CONTEMPLATIVE SCIENCE

COLUMBIA SERIES IN SCIENCE AND RELIGION

THE COLUMBIA SERIES IN SCIENCE AND RELIGION

The Columbia Series in Science and Religion is sponsored by the Center for the Study of Science and Religion (CSSR) at Columbia University. It is a forum for the examination of issues that lie at the boundary of these two complementary ways of comprehending the world and our place in it. By examining the intersections between one or more of the sciences and one or more religions, the CSSR hopes to stimulate dialogue and encourage understanding.

ROBERT POLLACK
The Faith of Biology and the Biology of Faith

B. ALAN WALLACE, ED.
Buddhism and Science: Breaking New Ground

LISA SIDERIS
Environmental Ethics, Ecological Theory, and Natural Selection: Suffering and Responsibility

WAYNE PROUDFOOT, ED.
William James and a Science of Religions: Reexperiencing The Varieties of Religious Experience

MORTIMER OSTOW
Spirit, Mind, and Brain: A Psychoanalytic Examination of Spirituality and Religion

B. ALAN WALLACE

CONTEMPLATIVE SCIENCE

WHERE BUDDHISM AND NEUROSCIENCE CONVERGE

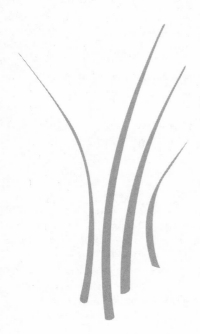

Columbia University Press

New York

COLUMBIA UNIVERSITY PRESS
Publishers Since 1893
New York   Chichester, West Sussex
Copyright © 2007 Columbia University Press

Library of Congress Cataloging-in-Publication Data
Wallace, B. Alan.
Contemplative science : where Buddhism and neuroscience converge / B. Alan Wallace
   p.   cm. — (The Columbia series in science and religion)
Includes bibliographical references and index.
ISBN 0–231–13834–2 (cloth : alk. paper) — ISBN 0–231–51095–0 (electronic)
1. Neurosciences—Religious aspects—Buddhism. 2. Buddhism—Psychology. I. Title. III.
   Series.
[DNLM: 1. Consciousness—physiology. 2. Neurosciences. 3. Buddhism. 4. Religion and
   Medicine.   WL 341 W187c 2007]
BQ4570.N48W35   2007
294.3'365—dc22
2006011012

Columbia University Press books are printed on permanent and durable acid-free paper.
This book was printed on paper with recycled content.
Printed in the United States of America
c 10 9 8 7 6 5 4

Designed by Lisa Hamm

CONTENTS

ACKNOWLEDGMENTS

I would first like to express my gratitude to Brian Hodel, who worked closely with me for months editing this series of essays into the present volume. Without his many editorial suggestions, from very specific aspects of the book to its general layout, this book likely would not have seen the light of day. My thanks also go to James Elliott, who helped to polish the manuscript, and to Wendy Lochner and Leslie Kriesel at Columbia University Press, for their invaluable role in producing this work.

I am indebted to the many fine scholars, contemplatives, and scientists who have inspired and critiqued this work, including Michel Bitbol, José Ignacio Cabezón, David Ritz Finkelstein, Owen Flanagan, Paul Gailey, Daniel Goleman, William Grassie, Charles L. Harper, Van Harvey, Anne Harrington, Piet Hut, David E. Meyer, Ken Paller, David Presti, Matthieu Ricard, Ben Shapiro, William Waldron, Zhihua Yao, and Arthur Zajonc. My understanding has been deeply enriched by all these individuals, and I am grateful for their collaboration.

I also wish to thank my parents for a lifetime of encouragement and good counsel, and my wife, Vesna A. Wallace, for her constant support and advice, which I seek at every turn. Finally, my boundless gratitude goes to all my teachers, particularly His Holiness the Dalai Lama, who have guided me in my pursuit of genuine happiness, truth, and virtue. I offer this book as a small token of thanks. May it be of benefit to others, as my teachers have benefited me.

He looked at his own Soul with a Telescope. What seemed all irregular, he saw and shewed to be beautiful Constellations: and he added to the Consciousness worlds within worlds.

—SAMUEL TAYLOR COLERIDGE

CONTEMPLATIVE SCIENCE

1

PRINCIPLES OF CONTEMPLATIVE SCIENCE

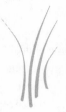 **THE VERY IDEA** of proposing a discipline called "contemplative science" may arouse suspicion among those who value the triumphs of science, which have been won, in part, by divorcing its mode of inquiry from all religious affiliations. Such unease has a strong historical basis, so it should be taken seriously. But there are also historical roots to the principles of contemplation and of science that suggest a possible reconciliation and even integration between the two approaches.

The Latin term *contemplatio*, from which "contemplation" is derived, corresponds to the Greek word *theoria*. Both refer to a total devotion to revealing, clarifying, and making manifest the nature of reality. Their focus is the pursuit of truth, and nothing less. As the Christian theologian Josef Pieper comments, the first element of the concept of contemplation is the silent perception of reality.[1] This, he claims, is a form of knowing arrived at not by thinking but by seeing. "Intuition is without doubt the perfect form of knowing. For intuition is knowledge of what is actually present; the parallel to seeing with the senses is exact."[2] But unlike objective knowledge, contemplation does not merely move toward its object; it already rests in it.

While the term "science" has long been affiliated solely with the exploration of objective, physical, quantitative phenomena—even to the point that they alone are deemed by some scientists to be real—there are also grounds for viewing science in a broader context. *Webster's Ninth New Collegiate Dictionary* defines the scientific method as follows: "Principles and procedures for the systematic pursuit of knowledge involving the recognition and formulation of a problem, the collection of data through observation and experiment, and the formulation and testing of hypotheses." There is nothing in this definition to preclude the possibility of first-person observations of mental phenomena and their relation to the world at large. Just as scientists make observations and conduct experiments with the aid of technology, contemplatives have long made their own observations and run experiments with the aid of enhanced attentional skills and the play of the imagination. In principle, then, there is nothing fundamentally incompatible between contemplation and science. But the weight of history is still against any fruitful collaboration between the two.

The strength science has acquired by divorcing itself from religion, and more recently from philosophy, has taken a severe toll on its host societies. It is sobering to note that the twentieth century, which generated the greatest growth of scientific knowledge in the entire course of human history, also witnessed man's greatest inhumanity to man, as well as the greatest degradation of our natural environment and the decimation of other species. The expansion of scientific knowledge has not brought about any comparable growth in ethics or virtue. Modern society has become more knowledgeable and powerful as a result, but it has not grown wiser or more compassionate.

Science has long been viewed proudly, not without justification, as being "value free." Time and again I have met with scientists who speak of the sheer joy of discovery, unrelated to any practical applications of their research. But we cannot ignore the fact that most scientific research is presently funded by governments and private institutions that have very specific goals in mind. They want a good return on their investments. With the modern dissolution of the medieval fusion of religion, philosophy, and science, there has occurred a similar disintegration of the pursuits of genuine happiness, truth, and virtue—three elements that are essential to a meaningful life. The contemplative science I have in mind seeks to reintegrate these three pursuits in a thoroughly empirical way, without dogmatic allegiance to any belief system, religious or otherwise. To explore this possibility, let us first review the salient features of genuine happiness, truth, and virtue that are to be united.

THE ESSENTIALS OF A MEANINGFUL LIFE

Genuine Happiness

Genuine happiness is a way of flourishing that underlies and suffuses all emotional states, embracing all the vicissitudes of life, and it is distinguished from "hedonic pleasure," which is the sense of well-being that arises in response to pleasurable stimuli. The Greek term that I am translating as genuine happiness is *eudaimonia*, which Aristotle in his *Nicomachean Ethics* equated with the human good. This is disclosed as a being-at-work of the soul in accordance with virtue, and if the virtues are more than one, in accordance with the best and most complete virtue.[3] Genuine happiness is not simply the culmination of a meaningful life, but a characteristic of a developing person in the process of ethical and spiritual maturation. This is an intentionally general notion of human flourishing that leaves it up to the individual reader to determine what virtues are "the best and most complete." Clearly, this ideal of genuine happiness can be embraced by both religious and nonreligious people, who may define its specific attributes in terms of their own worldviews. As we shall see in the following discussion, such well-being is a natural consequence of developing mental balance in ways that fortify the "psychological immune system," so that one rarely succumbs to a wide range of mental afflictions. A state of calm presence, emotional equilibrium, and clear intelligence are all characteristics of such genuine happiness, which naturally expresses itself in a harmonious, altruistic way of life.

Saint Augustine (354–430) raised this theme when he declared that the only thing we need to know is the answer to the question "How can man be happy?"[4] Genuine happiness, he declared, is a "truth-given joy,"[5] while the two real causes of the miseries of this life are "the profundity of ignorance" and the "love of things vain and noxious." The path to genuine happiness, he declared, is motivated by the love of God, which is the desire for union with him. This emphasis on the profundity of the pursuit of happiness is not confined to Greek antiquity or Christian theology. The Dalai Lama writes in his best-selling book *The Art of Happiness*, "I believe that the very purpose of our life is to seek happiness. Whether one believes in religion or not, whether one believes in this religion or that religion, we all are seeking something better in life. So, I think, the very motion of our life is towards happiness."[6]

Truth

Genuine happiness is not experienced simply as a result of encountering a pleasant sensory or intellectual stimulus. Nor is it produced merely by learning to think in a certain way or by adopting an optimistic attitude. It must be based on a sound understanding of truth. But there are many truths that have little relevance to human flourishing. Many of the aspects of the natural world studied by scientists seem far removed from human values, and there seems no reason to believe that scientists in general, for all their knowledge of the physical world, are happier than members of any other profession. As noted earlier, the exponential growth of scientific knowledge in the past century did not correspond to any comparable growth in human happiness, though advances in medicine have certainly contributed enormously to our physical well-being.

This implies that the types of truths most relevant to human flourishing are not those most commonly and successfully explored in modern science. While scientists have primarily focused their attention on the external world, there is no aspect of reality more pertinent to genuine happiness than the nature of human identity. Christian theologian Joseph Maréchal addresses this topic within the context of contemplative inquiry:[7]

> The human mind ... is a *faculty in quest of its intuition*—that is to say, of assimilation with Being, Being pure and simple, sovereignly one, without restriction, without distinction of essence and existence, of possible and real. ... But here below, in place of the *One*, it meets with the *manifold*, the *fragmentary*. Now, in the order of truth, the unreduced multiplicity of objects suspends affirmation and engenders doubt.... The affirmation of reality, then, is nothing else than the expression of the fundamental tendency of the mind to unification in and with the Absolute.

In the Buddhist tradition, as well, the importance of self-knowledge cannot be exaggerated, especially in light of the Buddhist assertion that the fundamental cause of human suffering is ignorance and delusion, specifically pertaining to one's own identity. Of all the virtues emphasized in Buddhism, none is more important than that of wisdom, entailing insight into the ultimate nature of reality. The seventh-century Indian Buddhist contemplative Śāntideva wrote, "The Sage taught this entire system for the sake of wisdom. Therefore, with the desire to ward off suffering, one should develop wisdom."[8]

Virtue

Just as genuine happiness is inextricably related to the understanding of truth, so it cannot be understood apart from virtue. While diverse theories of virtue abound among philosophers and theologians, Augustine's short definition is particularly salient and universal, as he explained it in terms of "the order of love," which has to do with the priority of our values.[9] Following the words of Jesus concerning the centrality of the love of God and of one's fellow humans, theologian John Burnaby writes, "The love of God which is the desire for union with Him, and the love of men which is the sense of unity with all those who are capable of sharing the love of God, are indeed bound up most intimately with one another."[10] This is the basis of all virtues within this theistic context.

In Buddhism, which is commonly referred to as a nontheistic religion, a life of virtue is a necessary foundation for pursuing truth and genuine happiness, or human flourishing, of which there are three kinds: social/environmental, psychological, and spiritual. While Buddhist theories of ethics are deeply embedded in the Buddhist worldview, including its assertions of reincarnation and karma, in his book *Ethics for the New Millennium* the Dalai Lama has developed a view of secular ethics that is equally relevant to religious believers and nonbelievers alike.

Psychological Flourishing

The explanatory power of behaviorism, psychology, and neuroscience pertains to topics such as decision making, attention, and statements about what subjects experience under various controlled conditions. The mental processes studied in the cognitive sciences consist largely of those that have, from an evolutionary perspective, helped mankind survive and procreate. All branches of psychophysics, attentional psychology, cognitive psychology, and personality and social psychology depend on asking people such questions as how bright something seems, what color they see, how loud they hear a sound, what they believe, what attitudes they have, and so on. Many of these data have been organized in terms of coherent principles, and the structured sets of findings that cognitive scientists have been trying to organize and understand are very large. Contemporary neuroscience has shed additional light on what psychologists have explored regarding memory, attention, emotions, attitudes, and so forth.

Especially since the Second World War, most psychological research, particularly in the United States, has been focused on normal and pathological mental processes. Only recently has scientific attention begun to focus on mental well-being, but funding for such research has been limited due to the fact that the nature of well-being and its behavioral effects are not well understood—a catch-22! This is where the contemplative traditions of the world, which have long been concerned with human flourishing within the context of truth and virtue, could make significant contributions.

Within the broad context of genuine happiness, it may be useful to identify specific domains of flourishing. On the basis of the social and environmental well-being that derives from the cultivation of ethical behavior, one may bring about psychological flourishing that emerges from a healthy, balanced psyche. I am using the word "psyche" to refer to the whole range of conscious and unconscious mental phenomena studied by psychologists, including perceptions of all kinds, thoughts, emotions, memories, fantasies, dreams, mental imagery, and so on. Psychological processes are conditioned by the body, personal history, the physical environment, and society, and from moment to moment they are closely correlated with specific brain functions. The psyche can be studied *indirectly* by the interrogation of individuals and by the examination of behavior and the brain, and it can be observed *directly* through introspection.

If psychological flourishing emerges from mental health and balance, it must be understood with respect to specific types of mental imbalances to which normal people—often deemed relatively healthy—are commonly prone. A fundamental premise behind the following analysis is that mental distress is generally a symptom of mental imbalances, much as physical pain is a symptom of physical illness or injury.[11] In the following sections, I shall set forth four kinds of mental imbalances—conative, attentional, cognitive, and affective—and for each one identify imbalances in terms of deficit, hyperactivity, and dysfunction.

Conative Imbalances

"Conation" is a valuable term, though not in common use, which refers to the faculties of desire and volition. Conative imbalances constitute ways in which our desires and intentions lead us away from psychological flourishing and into psychological distress. A conative deficit occurs when we experience an apathetic loss of desire for happiness and its causes and an unwillingness to alleviate our own and others' suffering. This is commonly accompanied by a lack of imagination and a kind of stagnated complacency: we can't imagine faring better, so we don't try to do anything to achieve such well-being. Conative hyperactivity occurs when we fixate on obsessive desires that obscure the reality of the present. We are so caught up in fantasies about the future—about unfulfilled desires—that our senses are dulled as to what is happening here and now. In the process, we may also blind ourselves to the needs and desires of others. Finally, conative dysfunction sets in when we desire things that are not conducive to our own or others' well-being, and don't desire the things that do contribute to our own and others' flourishing. It is crucial to recognize that individual psychological flourishing is not something that can be cultivated without any relation to others. We do not exist independently from others, so our well-being cannot arise independently of others either. We must take into account the well-being of those around us.

What kinds of goods (in the broadest sense, including both tangible and intangible things and qualities) are truly conducive to psychological flourishing? In his book *The High Price of Materialism*, psychologist Tim Kasser analyzes the relation between the materialistic values that so dominate today's world and the well-being that we all seek. He concludes:[12]

> Existing scientific research on the value of materialism yields clear and consistent findings. People who are highly focused on materialistic values have lower personal well-being and psychological health than those who believe that materialistic pursuits are relatively unimportant. These relationships have been documented in samples of people ranging from the wealthy to the poor, from teenagers to the elderly, and from Australians to South Koreans.

As noted earlier, Augustine pointed to the "love of things vain and noxious" as a kind of conative dysfunction, while the most profound, reality-based desire is the love of God, which is the desire for union with him. Nicholas of Cusa, a fifteenth-century cardinal of the Roman Catholic Church, echoed this theme when he wrote, "Everyone ... who is seeking seeks only the good and everyone who seeks the good and withdraws from you [God] withdraws from that which one is seeking."[13] Śāntideva expressed a similar theme from a nontheistic perspective: "Those seeking to escape from suffering hasten right toward their own misery. And with the very desire for happiness, out of delusion they destroy their own well-being as if it were their enemy."[14]

Although there are many ways of restoring conative balance, a general approach is to remedy apathy with the recognition of the possibility of genuine happiness, remedy obsessive desire with the cultivation of contentment, and remedy mistaken desires with the recognition of the true causes of genuine happiness and of our vulnerability to suffering. Specific methods for counteracting conative imbalances have been developed in various psychological and contemplative traditions for individuals committed to secular, theistic, and nontheistic worldviews.

Attentional Imbalances

No one who suffers from severe attentional imbalances can be deemed psychologically healthy. An attentional deficit is characterized by the inability to focus on a chosen object. The mind becomes withdrawn and disengaged, even from its own internal processes. Attentional hyperactivity occurs when the mind is excessively aroused, resulting in compulsive distraction and fragmentation. And attention is dysfunctional when we focus on things in afflictive ways, not conducive to our own or others' well-being. For example, a sex addict may attend to other people solely as sexual objects, and a salesperson may mentally engage with others only in terms of their willingness to buy a product. In such cases, the mind is prone to both attentional and conative imbalances, which often go hand in hand.

An attentional deficit corresponds closely to the Buddhist concept of laxity, and attentional hyperactivity correlates with excitation. These imbalances are remedied through the cultivation of mindfulness—the ability to sustain voluntary attention continuously upon a familiar object, without forgetfulness or distraction—and meta-attention—the ability to monitor the quality of the attention, swiftly recognizing whether it has succumbed to either excitation or laxity. Śāntideva emphasized the importance of developing attentional skills for psychological flourishing: "Upon developing zeal in that way, one should stabilize the mind in meditative concentration, since a person whose mind is distracted lives between the fangs of mental afflictions."[15]

While Buddhist contemplatives have identified and learned to heal these imbalances of the attention, the same issues have been of great concern to all the contemplative traditions of the world. An Eastern Orthodox Christian contemplative writes, "Keeping watch over his heart, growing in self-awareness, the aspirant acquires *nepsis* ('sobriety' or 'watchfulness') and *diakrisis* ('discernment' or 'discrimination,' the power to distinguish between good and evil thoughts)."[16] And Joseph Maréchal writes in a similar vein:

> There can be no contemplation without sustained attention, at least for a few moments; now attention acts on the psychological elements after the fashion of the poles of a magnet, which gather up iron filings into magnetic shapes. Perhaps the characteristic of contemplation is rather a deep *orientation* of the human being *in* an intuition or *towards* an intuition?[17]

Cognitive Imbalances

A person with a severe cognitive imbalance is radically out of touch with reality and is commonly diagnosed as suffering from some kind of psychosis. Normal people too are generally prone to cognitive imbalances, which lie at the root of much mental distress. Such imbalances are often deemed to be intrinsic to human nature, but this is an assumption that begs to be challenged by rigorous empirical inquiry.

Returning to the threefold analysis of mental imbalances, a cognitive deficit is characterized by the failure to perceive what is present in the five fields of sensory experience and in the mind. Insofar as we are out of touch with what is going on around us and within us, we are suffering from a cognitive deficit disorder. Cognitive hyperactivity sets in when we conflate our conceptual projections with actual perceptual experience—fail to distinguish between perceived realities and superimposed assumptions and fantasies. Psychotic people do this in extreme ways, while normal people are more discreet, but most of us are positioned on the same spectrum of cognitive hyperactivity, and it results in unnecessary mental suffering. Finally, cognitive dysfunction occurs when we misapprehend the way things are, through defects either in our physical senses or in our ability to interpret what is happening.

Overcoming such cognitive imbalance is a central theme in Buddhist practice, where one of the primary interventions is the cultivation of discerning mindfulness. The first challenge is to learn how to attend just to what is being presented to our senses and to inner awareness of our own mental processes. In this regard, the Buddha set forth the following ideal: "In the seen there is only the seen; in the heard, there is only the heard; in the sensed, there is only the sensed; in the mentally perceived, there is only the mentally perceived."[18] Elaborating on that theme, Buddhism gives detailed instructions on applying mindfulness to our own physical and mental presence in the world, with other beings, and with the inanimate environment. There is a rapidly growing mass of scientific research exploring the therapeutic effects of such mindfulness training, much of it inspired by the work of Jon Kabat-Zinn and his highly successful program of mindfulness-based stress reduction.

Affective Imbalances

Affective imbalances commonly occur as a result of conative, attentional, and cognitive imbalances, and they too can be viewed as being of three kinds. An affective deficit has the symptoms of emotional deadness within, and a sense of cold indifference toward others. Affective hyperactivity is characterized by alternating elation and depression, hope and fear, adulation and contempt, and obsessive craving and hostility. Affective dysfunction occurs when emotional responses are inappropriate to the circumstances at hand, such as taking delight in someone else's misfortune. Psychologists and contemplatives the world over have devised a wide array of interventions to heal such imbalances, some of them applicable to society in general, others embedded in religious worldviews. One fourfold approach drawn from Buddhism has spiritual depth without any necessary ties to a particular belief system. The essence of this practice is to remedy craving with loving-kindness, remedy aloof indifference with compassion, remedy depression with empathetic joy, and remedy personal prejudice with equanimity.

The overall effect of the four above-mentioned mental imbalances is constant dissatisfaction, which is only temporarily and superficially alleviated by latching onto pleasant sensory and mental stimuli or by altering the brain with drugs. Having little faith in their own inner resources for genuine happiness, many people today become addicted to pleasurable stimuli or chemical suppressants of dissatisfaction, but as soon as these props are removed, the sense of well-being disappears. From the perspective of contemplative science, the primary, pragmatic purpose of psychology is to explore states of the psyche to identify which lead to the perpetuation of suffering and which to genuine happiness. Like shifting from the use of fossil fuels to solar power, we have the opportunity to wean ourselves away from obsessive reliance on pleasurable stimuli and to shift to the cultivation of exceptional mental health as the basis of happiness.

A fundamental hypothesis behind this pursuit is that in terms of human nature, our habitual state is afflicted and suffering, but our potential state is healthy and flourishing. Our minds are not intrinsically unbalanced, only habitually so, and with continued, skillful effort, the imbalances may be remedied, resulting in a state of well-being that is not contingent upon agreeable sensory, chemical, intellectual, or aesthetic stimuli. This is an area in which science and the contemplative traditions may all collaborate for the benefit of the entire world.

There is a profound complementarity between scientific and contemplative approaches to the study of the psyche. The behavioral sciences, psychology, and neuroscience have shed light on cognitive processes that have enabled us to survive, propagate, and experience hedonic well-being. Contemplative traditions show how we can find genuine happiness, or eudaimonic well-being, and explore the spiritual dimensions of our existence. Hedonic and eudaimonic well-being do not usually stand in opposition to each other. On the contrary, without hedonic well-being, including good health and sufficient food, clothing, and shelter, it is difficult, though not impossible, to develop eudaimonic well-being. Likewise, the more we cultivate genuine happiness that arises from within, the more we can appreciate the simple pleasures of life. While hedonic well-being may have no intrinsic or enduring value, it can aid in seeking a meaningful life, entailing the integrated pursuit of genuine happiness, truth, and virtue.

THE ORIGINS OF THE PSYCHE

Contemporary cognitive scientists, confining their inquiries to behavior, brain activity, and the subjective reports of normal and subnormal people, have strongly held assumptions about the origins of the psyche: there is a widespread consensus that all mental processes are nothing more than functions or properties of the brain. And as long as scientific inquiry remains within those confines, it is unlikely that compelling evidence will emerge to seriously challenge that consensus. Scientific methods for studying the mind that are based on materialist assumptions will likely only reinforce them.

But Western philosophy and science did not always take such an attitude. Pythagoras (c. 570–c. 495 B.C.E.), the most famous of the pre-Socratic philosophers, who allegedly coined the term "philosophy," founded a contemplative community in the south of Italy that was both religious and scientific, with a strong emphasis on mathematics. Its main purpose was the cultivation of holiness through the purification of the body and mind. In his view, the man who devotes himself to such purification is the "true philosopher," one who "looks on" (*theorein*), and the greatest purification method of all is science.

Pythagoras is widely known for advocating a theory of metempsychosis, or reincarnation, according to which the soul is immortal and is reborn in both human and animal incarnations. This view was allegedly an empirical finding based on his own experience of recalling up to twenty of his own and others' past lives. The oldest and the latest accounts of his life agree in representing Pythagoras as a wonder worker, and the Pythagorean Society became the chief scientific school of ancient Greece.

In Plato's *Phaedo*, Socrates addressed this issue by first commenting that according to the popular view, the soul is dispersed and destroyed at death.[19] But the truth, he said, which is known only to those who have practiced philosophy, is far from that. The soul of the philosopher, having "practiced death" by shunning sensual craving and corporeal desires, "departs to a place which is, like itself, invisible, divine, immortal, and wise, where, on its arrival, happiness awaits it, and release from ... all ... human evils."[20] But the souls of those who have not practiced philosophy, being permeated by the corporeal, become wandering spirits after death, in a manner virtually identical to the

Buddhist account of the intermediate state (*antarābhava*) following death and prior to the next rebirth. Eventually, Socrates declared, "through craving for the corporeal, which unceasingly pursues them, they are imprisoned once more in a body. And as you might expect, they are attached to the same sort of character or nature which they have developed during life."[21]

Belief in metempsychosis was also common in early Christianity. Origen (185–254), widely viewed as the greatest Christian theologian after Paul and before Augustine, was strongly influenced by Pythagoras and Plato. Knowledge of God, he claimed, is natural to humanity and can be "recollected" and awakened by special disciplines. In this way, the soul can ascend to God in a long, steady journey from lifetime to lifetime. By means of contemplation (*theoria*), the soul advances in the knowledge (*gnosis*) of God, which transforms it until, as Plato had taught, it becomes divine. For Origen, like Pythagoras, there was no absolute divide between science and religion. The contemplative life may be subdivided into the contemplation of God and the contemplation of nature, and it has three stages: the active life (*praktikê*); the contemplation of nature, or "natural contemplation" (*physikê*); and contemplation in the strict sense, the vision of God, also termed "theology" (*theologia*), or "spiritual knowledge" (*gnosis*).[22] This unifying vision of science and spirituality was later suppressed when Emperor Justinian wrote a series of anathemas against Origen's writings. In the local synod of 543, he ordered the patriarch Mennas to call together all the bishops present in Constantinople and make them subscribe to the anathemas.

Despite the condemnation of Origen's writings concerning the origins of the soul, the matter was far from settled. Augustine addressed the issue by proposing four hypotheses: 1) an individual's soul derives from those of his or her parents; 2) individual souls are newly created from individual conditions at the time of conception; 3) souls exist elsewhere and are sent by God to inhabit human bodies; and 4) souls descend to the level of human existence by their own choice.[23] Augustine maintained that all these hypotheses are compatible with the Christian faith. In the true spirit of philosophy, he declared, "It is fitting that no one of the four be affirmed without good reason."[24] While many Christians today have chosen the second—that individual souls are newly created from individual conditions at the time of conception—the empirical and logical grounds for this view are far from clear.

The origins of the psyche were largely ignored by scientists from the time of Copernicus until the rise of modern psychology. William James, who founded the first neuroscience laboratory in the United States at Harvard University, proposed three hypotheses to explain the origins of mental processes in relation to brain functions: 1) the brain produces thoughts, as an electric circuit produces light; 2) the brain releases, or permits, mental events, as the trigger of a crossbow releases an arrow by removing the obstacle that holds the string; and 3) the brain transmits thoughts, as light hits a prism, thereby transmitting a spectrum of colors.[25] During his era and even today, all three of these hypotheses are consistent with everything that is scientifically known about mind-brain correlations. James, who believed in the third option, hypothesized:[26]

> When finally a brain stops acting altogether, or decays, that special stream of consciousness which it subserved will vanish entirely from this natural world. But the sphere of being that supplied the consciousness would still be intact; and in that more real world with which, even whilst here, it was continuous, the consciousness might, in ways unknown to us, continue still.

James further speculated that the stream of consciousness may be a different type of phenomenon than the brain, one that interacts with the brain while alive, absorbs and retains the identity, personality, and memories constitutive in this interaction, and can continue without the brain. While James is still widely respected among contemporary cognitive scientists, his views on the origins and nature of consciousness have been largely ignored or rejected. Most psychologists and neuroscientists categorically refute any kind of dualism on the ground that there is no evidence for the existence of any kind of subjective mental phenomenon apart from the functions and properties of the brain. But as long as cognitive scientists confine their inquiry to behavior, brain function, and the subjective reports of normal and pathological subjects, they have little chance of discovering evidence to the contrary.

One researcher who has scientifically challenged these views is Ian Stevenson, professor emeritus of psychiatry and the former director of the Division of Personality Studies at the University of Virginia.[27] In his recent book *Where Reincarnation and Biology Intersect*, he summarizes thirty years of research into alleged accounts of children accurately recalling specific people and events in their past lives. This book, written for the general public, consists mainly of abstracts of his studies, for which the detailed scientific accounts can be found in his massive, two-volume work *Reincarnation and Biology: A Contribution to the Etiology of Birthmarks and Birth Defects*. Stevenson's work provides some of the most compelling scientific evidence to challenge materialistic hypotheses about the origins of the psyche, but it has gone largely unnoticed by the scientific community.[28]

This refusal to examine empirical evidence that contradicts long-held beliefs has generally been more associated with religious believers than scientists. Physicist Richard Feynman poignantly expresses the scientific ideals of skepticism and empiricism: "Experimenters search most diligently, and with the greatest effort, in exactly those places where it seems most likely that we can prove our theories wrong. In other words we are trying to prove ourselves wrong as quickly as possible, because only in that way can we find progress."[29] Unfortunately, today's cognitive scientists do not seem eager to search in those places where their materialistic theories may be proved wrong. Insofar as their research pertains to the origins of the psyche, they seem single-mindedly committed to pursuing only those kinds of investigation that will reinforce their beliefs. To find viable alternatives to the scientific orthodoxy, we might best look outside of contemporary science to the world's contemplative traditions. I turn now to a Buddhist hypothesis that is based on contemplative training and is consistent with all that is currently known about brain-mind correlations.

The Substrate Consciousness

To discover the origins of any natural phenomenon, scientists have devised rigorous means of observing the phenomenon itself, conducting experiments on it when possible. This has been true for exploring the origins of all kinds of objects, from cells, on which experiments can be done, to stars, which can be observed but not manipulated through experimentation. The same is true for the psyche. To discover its origins, we must devise sophisticated methods for observing and experimenting on states of consciousness. It is not enough to observe and run experiments on their neural and behavioral correlates, and as long as cognitive science restricts its research to those, it cannot avoid the conclusion that consciousness emerges solely from the material processes under study. This is not a logical or empirical discovery, merely an inevitable conclusion based on a methodology of examining subjective, qualitative, mental processes by way of objective, quantitative, physical processes.

As a result of this orientation, cognitive scientists are confronted with an "explanatory gap": how is it that patterns of neural activity either produce or are equivalent to subjective mental processes? There are certainly kinds of neuronal activity that causally contribute to the emergence of specific states of consciousness and mental activity. Let's phenomenologically define causality as follows: if B follows A, and B does not occur in the absence of A, then A has a causal influence on B. No physical mechanism is necessarily required for a causal relation to occur, as has been amply demonstrated in electromagnetism and quantum mechanics. Philosopher John Searle argues that "lower order" neuronal activity "causes" mental processes, while "higher order" neuronal patterns are *equivalent* to mental processes.[30] Whether or not he's right, some kinds of prior neuronal activation are certainly necessary for the generation of specific, subsequent mental processes. But since those neural processes *precede* their resultant mental events, they can't be said to be *equivalent* to them. There could be an identity between only those neuronal and mental processes that occur simultaneously.

With regard to a causal relation between neural and mental events, we encounter philosopher David Chalmers's "hard problem":[31] what is it about those neuronal processes, unlike so many other electrochemical events, that enables them to produce the whole range of subjective mental experiences? Here is a serious explanatory gap. However, if certain neuronal processes are equated with their concurrent mental processes, what enables them to take on this dual nature: objective neuronal processes, which can be understood thoroughly in terms of physics, chemistry, and biology; and subjective mental processes that are undetectable using the instruments of measurement of these disciplines, but are immediately observable through first-person experience? It's as if these concurrent neuronal processes have a secret life that is hidden from third-person, scientific measurement: they are simultaneously objectively perceptible neural events and objectively invisible, subjective mental processes.

A simple fact that is hardly acknowledged by either cognitive scientists or philosophers of mind is that mental events *can* be observed directly. But, as James acknowledges, "Introspection is difficult and fallible; and ... the difficulty is simply that of all observation of whatever kind."[32] Crucial to making rigorous observations of mental phenomena is the cultivation of sustained, vivid, high-resolution attention, which Buddhists call *samādhi*. Such focused attention is to the scientific investigation of mental phenomena what the telescope is to the scientific investigation of celestial phenomena.[33] Buddhist contemplatives claim that with the achievement of a highly advanced degree of *samādhi* known as *śamatha*, or meditative quiescence, one gains experiential access to the relative ground state of consciousness known in the Great Perfection (Dzogchen) school of Tibetan Buddhism as the "substrate consciousness" (*ālayavijñāna*). This, they claim, is the individual stream of consciousness from which the psyche and all the physical senses emerge. According to their findings, the psyche is *conditioned* by the body and its physical interaction with the environment, but it *emerges* from the substrate consciousness.[34]

This is consistent with the hypotheses of Pythagoras, Socrates, Origen, Augustine, and William James, and it is compatible with everything that is currently known about mind-brain interactions. But this is also where all those contemplative views fundamentally diverge from the beliefs of most contemporary cognitive scientists. What Buddhism brings to this confrontation of worldviews is a practical way to put the hypothesis to the test of first-person experience, through the refinement of the attention and the settling of the mind in ways that are unknown to modern science.

One advantage of the cultivation of *śamatha* is that it does not require allegiance to any religious or philosophical belief system. Indeed, it has the potential to serve as a bridge between scientific and contemplative ways to explore the mind. When this exceptional degree of attentional balance is achieved, it is said that discursive thoughts become dormant and all appearances of oneself, others, one's body, and one's environment vanish. At that point, as in the states of sleeping and dying, the mind is drawn inward and the physical senses become dormant. Tibetan contemplatives report that what remains is a state of radiant, clear consciousness that is the basis for the emergence of all appearances to an individual's mind stream. All phenomena appearing to sensory and mental perception are imbued with the innate luminosity of this substrate consciousness. Like the reflections of the planets and stars in a pool of limpid, clear water, so do the appearances of the entire phenomenal world seem within this empty, clear, ground state of the psyche. Düdjom Lingpa (1835–1904), a Dzogchen master of the Nyingma order of Tibetan Buddhism, wrote, "The substrate consciousness, with its vacuous and clear nature, abides as the cause of everything that is emanated. The psyche that emanates from that substrate consciousness presents forms, which are stabilized by a continuous stream of consciousness."[35]

According to the experience of such contemplatives, there is a principle of conservation of consciousness that manifests in every moment of experience. The material constituents of the brain, such as neurons and electrochemical processes, do not transform into immaterial mental phenomena, such as dreams and hallucinations. No patterns of neuronal events actually *become* mental events. But nor do mental phenomena emerge from nothing. Rather, this empty, luminous, substrate consciousness transforms into the mental images, discursive thoughts, perceptions, emotions, and so on. In the course of a human life, these mental events are conditioned by the brain and environment, but they emerge from and dissolve back into the substrate consciousness. Likewise, these mental events *influence* the brain, body, and the physical environment, but they do not *transform into* those physical phenomena. In short, from this Buddhist perspective, the "hard problem" of how the brain produces subjective mental experience is a false problem, for such experience actually arises from the substrate consciousness. And the explanatory gap in demonstrating how some kinds of neural activity can be equivalent to mental events is unbridgeable, for neural and mental events are never identical.

The substrate consciousness may be characterized as a relative vacuum state, voided of all the "kinetic energy" of active thoughts, mental imagery, and sense perceptions. Generally speaking, it is indiscernible while the mind is active; it normally manifests only in dreamless sleep and at death. While the substrate consciousness is depicted as the natural, unencumbered state of the mind, its innate radiance and purity are present even when the mind is obscured by afflictive thoughts and emotions. When at rest, it is luminous and empty, but when catalyzed by thoughts or sensory stimulation, its "potential energy" transforms into the "kinetic energy" of the psyche, manifesting as all kinds of mental and sensory activity.

This dimension of individual consciousness transcends the specific qualities and limitations of personal history in this lifetime, gender, and even species, and this substrate underlies all forms of consciousness, human and nonhuman.[36] Once a contemplative's mind has settled in this silent, luminous state of awareness through the achievement of *śamatha*, it is said to be possible to direct the attention to the past, bringing to consciousness distinct, detailed memories of events that occurred years earlier in this lifetime. Then, through rigorous training, one may allegedly retrieve memories that precede the current life, remembering, like Pythagoras, the circumstances of preceding lives.

Such memories are not stored in the brain, though as long as the mind is *embodied*, the brain is necessary to retrieve them. Memories are stored, in a manner of speaking, in the continuum of the substrate consciousness, which carries on from lifetime to lifetime. This conclusion is based on the experiences of highly trained contemplatives who have refined their attention in ways unknown to modern science. Without such development of the internal telescope of *śamatha* for exploring deep states of consciousness, scientific evidence of reincarnation is limited to the field studies of researchers like Ian Stevenson.

While this description of the substrate consciousness may appear to be a Buddhist version of an immortal soul, it is important to note the differences between this experientially based account and various philosophical and theological speculations about the soul. Contemplatives who have achieved *śamatha* commonly depict this dimension of consciousness as a stream of arising and passing moments of awareness, so it is not a single entity persisting through time, nor is it unchanging. Moreover, it influences the psyche and is conditioned by physical and mental events, so it is not independent.

The substrate consciousness may be characterized as the relative ground state of the individual mind in the sense that within the context of an individual mind stream, it entails the lowest possible state of activity, with the highest possible potential and degree of freedom or possibility. For example, once an individual stream of consciousness has been aroused from dreamless sleep, it can freely manifest in a vast diversity of dreamscapes and experiences. Such exceptional creativity is displayed while under deep hypnosis, which also taps into the substrate consciousness. But this potential is most effectively accessed when one lucidly penetrates to the substrate consciousness by means of *śamatha*, as has been achieved in a number of the great contemplative traditions of the world. Śamatha entails vivid awareness of this dimension of consciousness, in contrast to the dullness that normally characterizes dreamless sleep.

Relative Vacuum States of Consciousness and of Space

The Great Perfection tradition of Tibetan Buddhism draws a distinction between the substrate consciousness (*ālayavijñāna*) and the substrate (*ālaya*), which is described as the objective, empty space of the mind and is subjectively experienced by the substrate consciousness. This vacuum state is immaterial, like space, a blank, unthinking void into which all objective appearances of the physical senses and mental activity dissolve when one falls asleep; and it is out of this vacuum that appearances reemerge upon waking. Düdjom Lingpa explained that when awareness settles in the substrate,

> the ordinary mind of an ordinary sentient being, as it were, disappears. Consequently, discursive thoughts become dormant, and roving thoughts vanish into the space of awareness.... Adhering to the experiences of vacuity and luminosity *while looking inwards*, the appearances of oneself, others, and objects vanish. That is the substrate consciousness ... one has come to the essential nature of the mind.[37]

This contemplative description of the substrate and the consciousness of that inner state of luminous vacuity is analogous to physicists' descriptions of the relative vacuum state of space. In general, a vacuum is defined as the lowest possible energy state of a volume of space, the result when everything else is taken away. The true, or absolute, vacuum consists of whatever remains once everything has been removed from some well-defined space— everything that the laws of nature permit. A false, or relative, vacuum consists of whatever remains once everything has been removed from some well-defined space that the current state of technology permits. The relative vacuum has energy and structure, and is not perfectly symmetrical, which is to say that it is internally differentiated.

Much as conscious appearances are said to emerge from the substrate and consist of configurations of this internal space of the mind, so do all configurations of mass and energy emerge from the vacuum and consist of configurations of physical space. Fields of elementary particles are nothing but excitations of empty space, and mass can be viewed as frozen energy. Light is a kind of excitation of empty space, or more accurately, an oscillation of abstract field quantities in space, not an oscillation of space proper. Physicist Henning Genz explains: "Real systems are, in this sense, 'excitations of the vacuum'—much as surface waves in a pond are excitations of the pond's water. ... The vacuum in itself is shapeless, but it may assume specific shapes. In doing so, it becomes a physical reality, a 'real world.'"[38]

While the vast majority of cognitive scientists today are convinced that the mind is nothing more than a function or emergent property of matter, physicists tells us that matter consists of oscillations of immaterial, abstract quantities in space. Further research is needed to determine whether these abstractions truly exist independently in objective space or are subjective artifacts of the minds that conceive them. Alternatively, the "real world" may be neither purely objective nor purely subjective.

William James's philosophy of radical empiricism closely reflects the view of the Great Perfection in rejecting the absolute duality of mind and matter in favor of a world of experience, in which consciousness *as an entity*, in and of itself, does not exist; nor is it a function of matter, for matter *as an entity*, in and of itself, does not exist either. According to this view, the ideas of mental and physical substances are conceptual constructs, as is the metaphysical distinction between subject and object. Mind and matter are constructs, whereas pure experience is primordial.

Absolute Vacuum States of Consciousness and of Space

In contrast to the substrate consciousness, which can be viewed as the relative ground state of the mind, according to the Great Perfection, primordial consciousness (*jñāna*) is characterized as the absolute ground state of consciousness. This state of perfect symmetry—internally undifferentiated in terms of any concepts or qualities—entails the lowest possible state of mental activity, with the highest possible potential and degree of freedom. While the substrate consciousness is aware of the substrate—the relative inner space of the mind—primordial consciousness is indivisibly aware of the absolute space of phenomena (*dharmadhātu*), which transcends the duality of external and internal space. All the phenomena that make up our intersubjective worlds of experience—appearances of external and internal space, time, matter, and consciousness—emerge from this absolute space and consist of nothing other than its configurations. In the limited, relative vacuum of the substrate, as in the case of deep sleep, mental events specific to one individual emerge and dissolve back into that subjective space of consciousness. But all phenomena throughout time and space emerge from and dissolve back into the timeless, infinite vacuum of absolute space. While the relative vacuum of the substrate can be ascertained by means of the cultivation of *śamatha*, the absolute space of phenomena can be realized only through the cultivation of contemplative insight (*vipaśyanā*).

The realization of absolute space by primordial consciousness transcends all distinctions of subject and object, mind and matter, indeed, all words and concepts. Such insight does not entail the meeting of a subjective mode of consciousness with an objective space, but rather the nondual realization of the intrinsic *unity* of absolute space and primordial consciousness. They are coterminous, nonlocal, and atemporal. While absolute space is the fundamental nature of the experienced world, primordial consciousness is the fundamental nature of the mind that experiences the world. But since the two have always been of the same nature, the view of the Great Perfection is not one of philosophical idealism, dualism, or materialism. All such distinctions between subject and object, mind and matter are regarded as mere conceptual fabrications. The indivisibility of absolute space and primordial consciousness is the Great Perfection, often referred to as the "one taste" of all phenomena.

On the relative level, the substrate consciousness is different from the substrate, and it is internally qualified by distinct experiences of bliss, luminosity, and nonconceptuality. It is experienced only when the mind is withdrawn from the external world, and it is bound by time and causality—specific to a given individual. The unity of absolute space and primordial consciousness, on the other hand, is also imbued with the qualities of bliss, luminosity, and nonconceptuality, not present as distinct attributes but as an ineffable unity.

This absolute vacuum is fathomed while letting consciousness come to rest in a state of nonduality, open to the entire universe. Devoid of all internal structure, it embodies a unique, absolute symmetry that transcends relative space, time, mind, and matter.

There are also important differences between the experiential effects of realizing the substrate consciousness and realizing primordial consciousness. When one realizes the substrate consciousness by achieving *śamatha*, mental afflictions are only temporarily suppressed, but it is said that by realizing primordial consciousness, all mental afflictions and obscurations can be eliminated forever. Likewise, the bliss that is experienced when resting in the relative ground state of consciousness is limited and transient, whereas the inconceivable bliss that is innate to the absolute ground state of primordial consciousness is limitless and eternal. By ascertaining the substrate consciousness, one realizes the relative nature of individual consciousness, but in the realization of primordial consciousness, the scope of awareness becomes boundless. Likewise, the creative potential of consciousness that is accessed through *śamatha* is limited, whereas that which is unveiled through such ultimate contemplative insight allegedly knows no bounds.

Primordial consciousness is said to be the ultimate source of genuine happiness, the ultimate truth that frees the mind of all afflictions and obscurations, and the ultimate wellspring of all virtue. It is in this dimension of consciousness that our deepest longing for happiness, truth, and virtue originates. This dimension is the alpha and omega of a meaningful existence, the ultimate ground of wisdom and compassion. The realization of primordial consciousness, when supported by the prior achievement of *śamatha*, is also said to open up limitless internal resources for various kinds of extrasensory perception and paranormal abilities. These include remote viewing, or clairvoyance; clairaudience; knowledge of others' minds; precognition; and other paranormal abilities, such as the ability to mentally control physical phenomena. Examples include moving through solid objects, walking on water, mental control of fire, flying, and mentally multiplying and transforming physical objects at will.

While claims of such seemingly miraculous, or supernatural, abilities are common in the annals of the contemplative traditions of the world, remote viewing and precognition have also been studied by modern researchers such as physicist Russell Targ.[39] The ability of the mind to influence physical objects has been studied by R. G. Jahn at the Princeton Engineering Anomalies Research Laboratory, but the findings of such researchers have been largely ignored by the scientific community. This may be due in part to the inconclusive results and to the inherently conservative nature of the scientific community, especially regarding alleged discoveries that undermine fundamental assumptions of the scientific worldview.

The research of Stevenson, Targ, and Jahn is like studying high-energy elementary particles by examining those that are occasionally and unpredictably produced in nature, whereas cultivating deep states of meditative concentration, or *samādhi*, is like building a particle accelerator so as to study high-energy particles under laboratory conditions. The many cognitive scientific laboratories for studying the brain and behavior may be well complemented by establishing laboratories for contemplative research, specifically designed to generate refined, "high-energy" states of awareness and use them to explore the potentials of consciousness and its role in the natural world.

Just as classical mechanics and engineering are useful for solving non-relativistic problems, the current cognitive sciences are useful for answering questions pertaining to normal and subnormal states of consciousness. But some of the underlying assumptions of classical physics have never been true, and some of the materialistic assumptions of classical cognitive science may prove to be equally untrue when exceptional states of consciousness are developed under controlled conditions and studied with scientific rigor.

The Buddhist description of the absolute space of phenomena bears some similarities to the absolute, or true, vacuum of modern physics. In 1973, Edward Tyron formulated the theory that the universe is one gigantic vacuum fluctuation with total energy equal to, or close to, zero. As Genz explains, "If its total energy equals or approximates zero, it may have originated as a spontaneous vacuum fluctuation. We might imagine that there is an approximate cancellation between the negative potential energies of all the masses that attract each other in the universe and the motion (or *kinetic*) and mass energies of these configurations."[40] Science writer K. C. Cole explains the symmetry of the true vacuum as follows:[41]

> If you can transform something such that the transformation doesn't make a noticeable difference, that's symmetry.... If something were *perfectly* symmetrical, then no matter how you tried to change it, the hypothetical change would have no effect. Without change, there is no perception. A perfectly symmetrical nothing would be a state so changeless that nothing you could conceivably do to it would make a difference.

Both the absolute space of phenomena and the true vacuum are said to have played a crucial role in formation of the universe as we know it. Henning Genz suggests,

Maybe quantum mechanical fluctuations initiated not only the *stuff* our world was made of prior to inflation but also space-time itself. Maybe the true *vacuum*, the true *nothing*, of philosophy and religion should be seen as a state wholly innocent of laws, space, and time. This state can be thought of as nothing but a collection of possibilities of what might be.[42]

K. C. Cole adds,

The release of energy may explain how the big bang got hot in the first place. Like water freezing into ice and releasing its energy into its surroundings, the "freezing" of the vacuum liberates enormous amounts of energy.... As simply as water freezing into ice, the inflated vacuum froze into the structure that gave rise to quarks, electrons, and eventually us.[43]

In a remarkably similar vein, the Dalai Lama writes in his recent book on the Great Perfection:[44]

Any given state of consciousness is permeated by the clear light of primordial awareness. However solid ice may be, it never loses its true nature, which is water. In the same way, even very obvious concepts are such that their "place," as it were, their final resting place, does not fall outside the expanse of primordial awareness. They arise within the expanse of primordial awareness and that is where they dissolve.

While physicists have devised their theories of the true and false vacuums on the basis of physical experiments and mathematical analysis, Buddhists have formulated their theories of true and false vacuum states of consciousness on the basis of contemplative experience and philosophical analysis. Both traditions place a high priority on empirical investigation and rational analysis, but their starting assumptions and modes of observation are profoundly different. The scientific revolution began with the assumption that an external God created the world prior to and independently of human consciousness. Physicists then set themselves the goal of perceiving that objective universe from a "God's-eye" perspective and formulating its laws in terms of God's own language, which they thought to be mathematics. Since they were focused on the realm of objective space and its contents that exist independently of consciousness, it was quite natural for them to marginalize the role of mind in nature; and their theories of the true and false vacuums generally make no reference to consciousness.

Indeed, advocates of this mechanistic view have assumed from the outset that consciousness plays no significant role in the universe. As neurologist

Antonio Damasio proclaims, "Understanding consciousness says little or nothing about the origins of the universe, the meaning of life, or the likely destiny of both."[45] Such confidence is remarkable in light of the fact that neuroscientists have not yet discovered the nature or origins of consciousness. Such researchers commonly assume that they already *know* that consciousness has no existence apart from the brain, so the only question to be solved is *how* the brain produces conscious states. In his book *The Discoverers: A History of Man's Search to Know His World and Himself*, historian Daniel J. Boorstin calls such assumptions "illusions of knowledge." It is these, he proposes, and not mere ignorance, that have historically acted as the greatest impediments to scientific discovery.[46]

The significance of the vacuum states of physical space and of consciousness can hardly be overestimated. Physicist John March-Russell declares, "The current belief is that you have to understand all the properties of the vacuum before you can understand anything else."[47] Physicists have not yet fathomed all the properties of the vacuum or all the laws of nature, but they have widely assumed that consciousness is irrelevant to the universe they are trying to understand. Insofar as the universe conceived by physicists exists independently of consciousness, Buddhists may counter that such a universe is irrelevant to the world of human experience, in which consciousness plays a crucial role.

Convergence with Christianity

While the scientific revolution was deeply influenced by the belief in a God who exists absolutely outside of his creation and who observes and rules the world from an absolutely objective perspective, this is not the only theology that has been advocated by devout Christians through the ages. In contrast to the pursuit of a God's-eye view that has so influenced modern science, Eastern Orthodox Christian contemplatives have long advocated a kind of natural contemplation of seeing God in all things and all things in God, to discern the divine presence that is within each natural phenomenon and at the same time transcends it. The emphasis is on the immanence of God, instead of solely on his transcendence. Rather than seeking to comprehend the world using the language of mathematics, these contemplatives have sought to know God by moving beyond all kinds of thought and language:[48]

> Since the deity is a mystery beyond words and understanding, it follows that in such contemplation the human mind has to rise above concepts, words, and im-

ages—above the level of discursive thinking—so as to apprehend God intuitively through simple "gazing" or "touching." As Evagrius put it, the mind is to become "naked," passing beyond multiplicity to unity.... At the higher levels of contemplation, then, awareness of the subject-object differentiation recedes, and in its place there is only a sense of all-embracing unity.

Rather than regarding the God's-eye view as being absolutely external to the human mind, Neo-Platonic Christian contemplatives following the tradition of the ninth-century Christian translator and philosopher John Scotus Eriugena (815?–877?) saw the possibility of seeking God within oneself. Nicholas of Cusa, who belonged to that contemplative tradition, likewise believed that the face of God can be known only by transcending all concepts, including mathematical ones. By so doing, he claimed, one may achieve "absolute sight, the source of all the sight of those who see, [that] excels all sharpness, all quickness, and all power of all who actually see and all who can become seeing."[49]

According to the Great Perfection tradition, ordinary, dualistic perception could not exist in the absence of primordial consciousness, and Nicholas of Cusa expressed a similar view when he declared, "Without absolute sight there can be no contracted sight. Sight that is absolute embraces in itself all modes of seeing, and it embraces all modes in such a way as to embrace each, and it remains entirely absolute of every variety."[50] And he made another remarkable claim similar to the Buddhist assertion that the whole of reality can be fathomed by comprehending the nature of consciousness: "Whoever, therefore, merits to see your face sees all things openly and nothing remains hidden to this person."[51] Indeed, many of the great Christian mystics, including Augustine, have declared that an effect of their contemplative practice was a clearer perception of the nature of God, the human soul, and the laws of nature.[52]

Some of the Christian contemplative insights into the nature of the material world seem to lend credence to this assertion. Material phenomena that appear to make up our physical environment, according to Nicholas, consist of "contracted natures," and the same is true of ordinary mental phenomena. This theme appears in principle to be remarkably similar to the metaphor of ordinary states of matter and consciousness existing as "frozen" manifestations of the ultimate nature of reality. Nicholas writes in a similar vein, "prime matter's power to be is material and thus contracted and not absolute; so too sensible or rational power to be is contracted, but completely uncontracted power coincides with the simply absolute, that is, with the infinite."[53] According to modern physics, the absolute vacuum has the unique characteristic of perfect symmetry, as does the absolute space of phenomena, according to the Great Perfection view. And Nicholas commented, "All things that are said of God cannot differ in reality because of God's highest simplicity."[54] The ultimate theme of the Great Perfection is the nonduality of relative and absolute dimensions of reality, a belief with which Nicholas seems to concur: "There is nothing outside you, but all things in you are not other than you. You teach me, Lord, how otherness, which is not in you, does not exist in itself, nor can it exist."[55]

The above, brief discussion is obviously not conclusive. There are many important differences between Buddhist and Christian theories of consciousness, and between scientific and contemplative theories of space. But in the midst of these doctrinal and theoretical differences, there may also be a common, hidden ground on which these diverse traditions ultimately converge. If so, I believe they are converging on the most important truth that can be known and experienced. This is the truth that yields genuine happiness and results in a life of virtue in service to all beings.

CHALLENGES FOR A CONTEMPLATIVE SCIENCE

A central challenge facing contemplative science is to naturalize consciousness without reducing it to an emergent property or a function of matter. This requires exploring alternatives other than Cartesian dualism, which has proven futile, and scientific materialism, which severely limits our understanding of the nature and potentials of consciousness.

We are also faced with the challenge of fundamentally reassessing human nature. If we rely solely on physics to understand our place in nature, human existence is reduced to the status of a robot. If we rely solely on biology, we are reduced to the status of animals. Contemporary, mainstream psychology has largely confined itself to the study of normal and subnormal human minds, and has defined human identity within those limitations. Buddhism views our existence in terms of three dimensions: human nature qualified by the human body and psyche, and our nature as sentient beings, qualified by the individual substrate consciousness and by primordial consciousness, which transcends all limitations of individual human or sentient existence. Christianity declares that man is created in the image of God, which gives a basis for Jesus' challenge for each person to be perfect as the Father in heaven is perfect. But it also depicts human nature as fallen and therefore in need of redemption through Christ.

In terms of our view of reality as a whole, I have argued that the underlying principles of modern science are valid with respect to the objective physical world devoid of subjective awareness, and as long as one ignores the implications of refining consciousness (e.g., through the cultivation of *samādhi*). This neglect of the role of consciousness can seem insignificant, much as the underlying assumptions of classical mechanics appear valid as long as the matter being studied is large and doesn't approach the speed of light. But when consciousness is highly refined, it becomes necessary to speak of "relativistic" states of consciousness (so called, because their relevance to the physical world becomes obvious); current materialistic assumptions may prove to be false.

The contemplative refinement of consciousness and the scientific investigation of the implications of such states of consciousness may explicitly revolutionize the cognitive sciences and implicitly revolutionize natural science as a whole, which is largely based on the assumptions of nineteenth-century materialism. This will require a thorough investigation of the causal efficacy of consciousness, especially relativistic states of consciousness, in the natural world. This, in turn, may bring forth a science of the world of experience that replaces our current science of a purely objective world, devoid of subjectivity.

The ideals of the contemplative life have almost vanished in the modern West, but we need not look outside our culture to rediscover them. Indeed, we need look no further than Thomas Aquinas, whose influence on Western Christianity can hardly be overestimated: "It is requisite for the good of the human community that there should be persons who devote themselves to the life of contemplation."[56] The very purpose of civilization is the pursuit of genuine happiness, truth, and virtue, and the contemplative life is entirely focused on these themes. This, I believe, is what Aquinas had in mind when he wrote:[57]

> The whole of political life seems to be ordered with a view to attaining the happiness of contemplation. For peace, which is established and preserved by virtue of political activity, places man in a position to devote himself to contemplation of the truth.

2

WHERE SCIENCE AND RELIGION COLLIDE

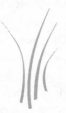 **IN THE AMERICAN** educational system and the general media, science is commonly presented as a body of empirical knowledge about the natural world, discovered by researchers who are relentlessly skeptical of all untested assumptions and beliefs, including their own. Religions, in contrast, are often presented as promoting beliefs about the universe and the meaning of human existence that are accepted by their adherents on the basis of divine authority. Thus, science and religion appear to stand for two incompatible mind-sets, and conflict between these two ways of viewing reality seems inevitable.

While there is some truth in this depiction, in many ways it is profoundly misleading and has resulted in widespread confusion about the nature of both science and religion. Science as a method of inquiry has been an extremely powerful tool for investigating the nature of the universe, and it has provided deep insights that have changed human perspectives and lives throughout the world. But the success of the scientific approach has led to speculative extensions of its findings into areas of metaphysics where in fact there is no experimental evidence one way or another. This is the genesis of scientific materialism, which is a dogma, not a scientific theory. Uncritical adherence to this system of belief does a great disservice to science itself, because it creates confusion about the real nature, power, and limitations of scientific inquiry. And it is dangerous for society, because if the state accepts without question a metaphysical system that focuses exclusively on material issues, human existence is impoverished and the way is open for the kinds of environmental and personal degradation that plague modern life.

The scientific materialist worldview may be summed up as follows: the physical world is the only reality. It originates wholly from impersonal natural forces; it is devoid of any intrinsic moral order or values; and it functions without the intervention of immaterial spiritual forces of any kind, benevolent or otherwise. Life and consciousness originally arose in this universe purely by accident, from complex configurations of matter and energy. Life in general, and human life in particular, has no meaning, value, or significance other than what it attributes to itself. During the course of an individual's life, all desires, hopes, intentions, feelings, and so forth—in short, all experiences and actions—are determined solely by the body and the impersonal forces acting upon it from the physical environment. The termination of an individual's life results in the disappearance of consciousness and the utter annihilation of the individual, and eventually this is the destiny of all life in the universe: it will simply disappear without a trace. In short, man is fundamentally isolated; he lives on the boundary of an alien world, which is as indifferent to his hopes as it is to his suffering or his crimes. Only by accepting this view of human existence and the universe at large can humans live authentically.

Science has always evolved in close interaction with the prevailing religions and philosophies of its host cultures. The above perspective is closely linked to the materialist ideology of Marx, which filtered into science through such figures as the Russian Marxist Aleksandr Oparin, who in 1938 published an influential book proposing that life originates from nonlife, implying a smooth continuum from inorganic to organic matter.[1] One can also see in the above depiction of the universe close parallels to the twentieth-century existentialism of Sartre and Camus, and reflections of the ethical relativism of postmodernists such as Derrida and Foucault. But philosophy is philosophy. Let us not confuse it with empirical science.

Scientific materialism is incompatible with all the major world religions, and it has been presented as scientific knowledge by many prominent scientists, including Carl Sagan, Richard Feynman, Jacques Monod, Richard Dawkins, Francis Crick, Edward O. Wilson, Steven Weinberg, Stephen Jay Gould, and Antonio Damasio, to name several. Methodologically, it is quite reasonable for science to adopt the working hypotheses of naturalism, that is, to seek to understand the world in terms of natural, not supernatural agencies. Scientific theories, in contrast to philosophical ideas and religious beliefs, must be submitted to empirical observation and experimentation. But scientific materialists commonly take the further step of promoting a worldview that makes claims that go beyond the scope of scientific knowledge.

Contrary to the position of many ardent scientific materialists, belief in this worldview is not necessary for practicing excellent science. It is merely a secondary opinion that some scientists have about existence. Belief is central to both science and religion, but it usually plays a different role in each context. In science, the beliefs that are brought into research and teaching act as a set of working hypotheses. These are not meant to be dogmatic, but rather to be assumptions that allow scientists to ask particular questions. Ideally, all of these assumptions are subject to empirical refutation. Working hypotheses can be accepted for the purpose of attempting to make progress in science, but they must be tentative as well, even if some of them are taken as "facts." By their own standards of skepticism, scientists must be open-minded enough to recognize that any of these hypotheses could ultimately be discarded.

Over time, however, working hypotheses can easily transform into closely held beliefs, and it is here that dogma creeps in. The term "dogma" refers to a coherent, universally applied worldview consisting of a collection of beliefs and attitudes that call for intellectual and emotional allegiance. As such, a dogma has a power over individuals and communities that is far greater than the power of mere facts and fact-related theories. Indeed, it may prevail despite the most obvious contrary evidence, and commitment to it may grow all the more zealous when obstacles are met. There are many kinds of dogmas, including religious, philosophical, political, and scientific.

It is commonplace to ignore evidence that conflicts with scientists' most fundamental working hypotheses. For all its emphasis on the ideal of skepticism, science is conservative, and a paradigm shift doesn't happen easily. In that sense, dogma can be conceived of as relative rather than absolute. On the one hand, doing science entails taking many assumptions as beliefs, to varying extents. On the other hand, scientific inquiry is conducted by people, and people are governed by various forces—political, sociological, and others—so the ideals of science may be quite different from its actual practice.

THE DOGMA OF SCIENTIFIC MATERIALISM

Scientists are no freer of dogma than are politicians, philosophers, or theologians. It can be argued, however, that there is a subtle but important difference between the closely held beliefs of scientists and nonscientists. The beauty and wonder of science is that it has been growing over twelve generations in a way that is far more open and accepting of change than almost all individual scientists are. Scientists are limited human beings, but science as a method seems to transcend many of the limitations of its practitioners. Hence the common saying that an older generation of scientists has to die off to make room for new ideas, since many individuals cannot fully accept radical new insights. Given all this, it may well be that, with enough time, current scientific dogmas will eventually be challenged and perhaps overturned. This depends, though, on future societies and cultures living long enough and with sufficient freedom of inquiry to let science continue. Research that challenges the dogmas of science must be not only tolerated but also encouraged.

I turn now to a closer examination of the essential principles of the ideology of scientific materialism.

Objectivism

The principle of objectivism requires that science deal with empirical facts testable by empirical methods and verifiable by third-person means. The phenomena that best lend themselves to such inquiry are universal, public, controlled, repeatable, and predictable. In the minds of some scientific materialists, the affirmation of scientific objectivism also implies a commitment to the view that, in the words of sociobiologist Edward O. Wilson, "Outside our heads there is freestanding reality.... Inside our heads is a reconstitution of reality based on sensory input and the self-assembly of concepts."[2] The proper task of scientists, he claims, is to correctly align the subjective representation of reality inside our heads with the objective, external world. This view, which is rooted in the seventeenth-century metaphysics of René Descartes, implies that the objective world *lies beyond* the subjective world of appearances, including all the evidence from our senses, which are deemed to exist only within our heads.

Reductionism

While there are various kinds of reductionism, "categorical reductionism" is the tendency to reduce something relatively unfamiliar or poorly understood to a more familiar and understood class of phenomena. While this has always been a general psychological method for acquiring understanding of the world, due to the specific sequence of the development of the major branches of natural science, reductionism in science has taken on a special orientation. Historically, the physical sciences made the first great advances and established what has come to be known as the scientific method, so it was natural for later generations of biologists to try to understand living organisms in terms of physics. Physicist Richard Feynman expressed this view when he declared in an undergraduate course, "There is nothing that living beings do that cannot be understood from the point of view that they are made of atoms acting according to the laws of physics."[3] Cognitive scientists, in turn, try to understand mental processes in terms of the biological mechanisms of the brain and of artificial intelligence systems. Likewise, academic scholars of religion commonly seek to explain spiritual experiences in terms of psychology, medicine, economics, and other nonreligious factors.

Nowhere is such categorical reductionism more commonly applied than to the study of human behavior and the mind, two of the most mysterious and complex fields of scientific inquiry. Biologist Richard Dawkins, for instance, claims that genes are the central evolutionary driver and that human beings, like all animals, are basically machines created by our genes. Writing about genes as if they had conscious aims, he posits that they control human behavior, "not directly with their fingers on puppet strings, but indirectly like the computer programmer."[4] In the same spirit of categorical reductionism, neurologist Antonio Damasio declares,

> Many of us in neuroscience are guided by one goal and one hope: to provide, eventually, a comprehensive explanation for how the sort of neural pattern that we can currently describe with the tools of neurobiology, from molecules to systems, ever becomes the multidimensional, space-and-time-integrated image we are experiencing this very moment.[5]

As a research strategy, reductionism has proved its pragmatic value countless times in the history of science. Some scientists cautiously embrace reductionism as a *method* that has proven highly useful in many areas of research, without adopting it as a *belief* about the actual nature of reality as a whole. But even as a method, it has its limits. Biologists, for example, know that they cannot explain such things as animal behavior in terms of the individual movements of molecules; and cognitive scientists are aware that complex mental processes cannot be understood in terms of the behavior of individual neurons.

The Closure Principle

The closure principle declares that even if nonmaterial phenomena do exist, they never exert any influences within the physical universe. That is, the universe is closed off from any hypothetical nonphysical causal agents. Adopting this principle as a working hypothesis makes perfectly good sense when the tools of research are confined to the measurement of physical phenomena. But the implications of this principle, inflated to a metaphysical statement of fact, are enormous, in terms of both the boundaries of scientific knowledge and the nature of human existence. In his book *The Blind Watchmaker,* Richard Dawkins transcends the legitimate domain of science when he claims:

> Natural selection, the blind, unconscious, automatic process which Darwin discovered, and which we now know is the explanation for the existence and apparently purposeful form of all life, has no purpose in mind. It has no mind and no mind's eye. It does not plan for the future. It has no vision, no foresight, no sight at all. If it can be said to play the role of watchmaker in nature, it is the *blind* watchmaker.[6]

Physicist Steven Weinberg makes the same error in the oft-quoted statement in his book *The First Three Minutes*: "The more the universe seems comprehensible, the more it also seems pointless."[7] It is not that scientific materialists don't like to address metaphysical issues. They do, but they often misrepresent them as scientific conclusions. In this way they do a great disservice to understanding both science and religion.

Physicalism

The principle of physicalism declares that the universe consists solely of configurations of matter and energy within space and time. To understand this principle, it is crucial to recognize that the matter in question is not the familiar stuff that we bump into in everyday experience. A rock held in the hand, for instance, is experienced as having a certain color, texture, and weight. But all those qualities are *secondary attributes* that exist, according to a line of thinking tracing back to Descartes, not in the objective world but as representations inside our heads. The matter that constitutes the fundamental building blocks of the objective universe, according to scientific materialism, exists prior to and separate from all such secondary attributes that arise only in relation to a conscious subject. The real properties of matter are its inherent, *primary attributes* that exist independently of all modes of detection.

HOW WELL DOES SCIENTIFIC MATERIALISM WORK?

One of the most common arguments in support of regarding the principles of scientific materialism as scientific knowledge is that they *work*. That is, pragmatically speaking, they have proven to be extremely useful. A second argument in support of their validity is that no evidence has ever been found to refute them. If those two assertions are true, then we must take seriously the hypothesis that the adoption of those principles is necessary for conducting any kind of scientific research. Let us therefore turn to an evaluation of scientific materialism in terms of its pragmatic value and its validity.

Objectivism and the Cognitive Sciences

In its emphasis on the scientific study of universal, public, controlled, repeatable, and predictable phenomena, the principle of objectivism marginalizes all that is individual, private, uncontrolled, unique, and anomalous. This accounts in large part for the fact that the scientific study of the mind did not even begin until three hundred years after the beginning of the scientific revolution. But such phenomena, including all kinds of subjective mental processes, are no less real or significant than those that measure up to the principle of objectivism. Prioritizing the reality and significance of purely objective phenomena devalues subjective experience to such an extent that it is commonly regarded as a mere epiphenomenon of the objective physical processes that "underlie" it.

This bias, which dominated the school of behaviorism begun in the early twentieth century by John B. Watson, has marginalized first-person, introspective ways of examining mental phenomena. Indeed, Watson went so far as to declare that behaviorists must exclude from their scientific vocabulary "all subjective terms such as sensation, perception, image, desire, purpose, and even thinking and emotion as they are subjectively defined."[8] Regarding subjective mental events as nonexistent, purely on dogmatic grounds, can hardly be a pragmatically useful principle for understanding such events. Only recently have cognitive scientists begun to reconsider that introspection may play a valuable role in studying conscious mental phenomena and that subjective experience does influence brain functions. Adherence to the dogma of scientific materialism has blinded scientists from seeing these truths, which have long been evident to nonscientists.

The legitimate domain of scientific inquiry, according to the principle of objectivism, is the objective world, which exists independently of anyone's mind. Pragmatically speaking, phenomena are deemed "objective" when they are broadly intersubjective; that is, they are apprehended by a wide range of subjects using different modes of observation. Everything of which we are conscious appears in relation to our faculties of sensory and mental perception. We have no direct knowledge of anything that exists independently of consciousness. Physicist Werner Heisenberg commented, "What we observe is not nature in itself but nature exposed to our method of questioning."[9] And Albert Einstein commented in a similar vein, "On principle, it is quite wrong to try founding a theory on observable magnitudes alone. In reality the very opposite happens. It is the theory which decides what we can observe."[10]

As an ardent scientific materialist, Wilson claims that this objectivist worldview is empirical, radically unlike the transcendentalism of religion. At the same time, he rightly acknowledges there is no objective yardstick on which to mark the degree of correspondence between the physical world and mental representations. This ironically implies that the real, objective world that he claims is the proper domain of science transcends all empirical data and can be known only indirectly, by way of subjective, mental representations. So scientific materialists like Wilson are actually advocating their own version of transcendentalism with respect to the very existence of the objective world that they seek to understand.

Reductionism, the Closure Principle, and the Life Sciences

While there are obvious advantages to explaining novel phenomena in terms of more familiar phenomena, this tendency can also have disadvantages: such reductionism may obscure the unique qualities of things that are significantly unlike others better known. As mentioned previously, among the various branches of natural science, the physical sciences became the model for the life sciences and the cognitive sciences that developed thereafter. While there is a strong tendency to try to reduce cognitive processes to biological processes and biological processes to inorganic physical processes, it turns out that there is a hierarchy among these three branches of science.

The explanations of the physical sciences are necessary but not sufficient for understanding biological processes. That is, there is nothing in the laws of physics that predicts the emergence of life in the universe. And if physicists were to confine their research to the theoretical and empirical methods of physics alone, ignoring all that has been learned from the life sciences, they could neither define nor empirically detect the presence of living organisms. Likewise, the explanations of the biological sciences are necessary but not sufficient for understanding mental processes. Once again, there is nothing in the laws of biology or evolution that predicts the emergence of subjective mental phenomena in the universe. And if biologists were to confine their research to the theoretical and empirical methods of biology alone, ignoring all that has been learned from psychology, they could neither define nor empirically detect mental phenomena. Following this same theme, it may well be that explanations of the cognitive sciences are necessary but not sufficient for understanding spiritual experiences. There is certainly nothing in the cognitive sciences to predict their occurrence, and cognitive scientists can neither define nor empirically detect spiritual experiences without relying on the first-person accounts of people who have them.

By adhering to the principle of reductionism, with physics underlying biology and biology underlying psychology, scientific materialists have long assumed that the physical sciences have nothing to learn from the life sciences, the life sciences have nothing to learn from psychology, and psychology has nothing to learn from religion. But given the hierarchy among the natural sciences outlined above, it may be time to apply a healthy dose of scientific skepticism to this metaphysical claim.

Before leaving the topic of reductionism, it may be useful to review its applicability with regard to the scientific understanding of evolution, which provides great insights into the ways living organisms survive and procreate. If the human brain and sensory system evolved as a biological apparatus to preserve and multiply human genes, as Richard Dawkins maintains, how is it that we humans have the capacity to experience universal love and concern for the welfare of the human race as a whole? As Dawkins admits, such facts "simply do not make evolutionary sense."[11]

Humans are concerned not only with survival and procreation but also with the pursuit of meaning and happiness. But meaning, Wilson writes, "is the linkage among the neural networks created by the spreading excitation that enlarges imagery and engages emotion."[12] While the subjective sense of meaning undoubtedly has neural correlates, to reduce this crucial feature of human existence to brain chemistry is to miss the point entirely. The nature of a meaningful life is not explained by such reductionism, any more than the beauty of the Mona Lisa is explained by the chemical composition of its paint. Likewise, concerning the pursuit of happiness, Wilson acknowledges that millions seek it and "feel otherwise lost, adrift in a life without ultimate meaning," but he suspects that it will eventually be explained as "brain circuitry and deep, genetic history."[13] Scientific materialism offers no clue as to how humans might actually experience genuine happiness, for this is one more facet of human existence that does not make "evolutionary sense."

The principle of reductionism and the closure principle also have great ramifications for the question of free will. If there is such a thing as freedom

of the will, there must be someone to exert that freedom, to make free deci-
sions. Wilson responds, "Who or what within the brain monitors all this
activity? No one. Nothing. The scenarios are not seen by some other part of
the brain. They just *are*."[14] If there is no individual identity or self apart from
brain function, the question of free will seems moot. But Wilson doesn't leave
it there. The hidden, cerebral preparation of mental activity, he claims, gives
the *illusion* of free will. The fact that it is an illusion, he claims, is bolstered by
the ungraspable complexity of the material influences on the brain. In short,
according to scientific materialism, our very survival depends in part upon
the maintenance of the illusion of free will. But if this is true, and, as scientific materialism has argued, we do not even exist as individuals who make
real choices, it would follow that the proliferation of scientific materialism is
undermining our very chances of survival as a race. For once an illusion is
unveiled—for example, when a child is told that Santa Claus doesn't really
exist—its ability to influence the course of our lives is undermined.

The theory of evolution is one of the most important achievements of
modern science, but when it is bound by the metaphysical constraints of
reductionism and the closure principle, it not only fails to account for many
important features of human existence but also makes them unintelligible.

Physicalism and the Physical Sciences

The physical sciences were developed to measure and explain only physical phenomena, but the metaphysical principle of physicalism declares that
everything consists of configurations of matter and energy and their emergent properties within space and time. Physicists agree that matter consists
of atoms, which in turn are made up of elementary particles such as electrons and protons. Then, according to some leading physicists, elementary
particles are composed of strings existing in eleven dimensions.[15] Operationally, there is a wide consensus as to ways of measuring physical phenomena and the quantitative laws that govern their interactions. But the actual
nature of these fundamental building blocks of the universe as they exist
independently of all measurements in the objective world is shrouded in
mystery. Some physicists argue that atoms are nothing more than properties
of space-time, but the very concept of space-time and its dimensions isn't
precisely defined. Others maintain that atoms are not things at all, but are
better viewed as sets of relationships.

In terms of quantum mechanics, it appears increasingly dubious whether
the elementary particles of matter have any discrete location independent of

all systems of measurement. Experts have expressed diverse views ranging from the assertion that elementary particles exist independently as real, distinct entities to the view that there is no objectively existing quantum realm at all! As physics continues to progress, the primary status of matter becomes increasingly elusive. Physicist Steven Weinberg goes so far as to proclaim, "In the physicist's recipe for the world, the list of ingredients no longer includes particles. Matter thus loses its central role in physics. All that is left are principles of symmetry."[16]

Upon confronting such startling lack of consensus about the nature and primacy of matter, scientific materialists may take refuge in the notion of energy and its conservation as the primary stuff of the universe. But this provides little consolation, for according to Richard Feynman, the conservation of energy is a mathematical principle, not a description of a mechanism or anything concrete. He then goes on to acknowledge, "It is important to realize that in physics today we have no knowledge of what energy is."[17]

The material world is much more complex from a scientific perspective, as understood today, than scientific materialists can hope to grasp with their simple metaphysics, rooted in the seventeenth-century mechanistic view of reality. It seems that matter presently fills the role for the advocates of this metaphysical dogma that God has traditionally filled for the theist. But the diverse speculative theories of these "materialogians" provide little support for the belief that such mysterious stuff can support the ontological burden of the entire universe of subjective and objective phenomena.

The role that matter plays in scientific materialism in the sense of "holding up" things is far different from the role it currently plays in physics, where "matter" refers to the mysterious counterpart of scientific mathematical theories. What counts in physics is to get the theories right, and to test them against observations. Most physicists don't any longer ask additional questions, such as what matter really is; such inquiries are viewed as irrelevant. But if physicists no longer claim to know what matter or energy is, the metaphysical assertion that everything in the universe can be reduced to matter and its emergent properties has to be reappraised. Rather than an *ontological* reduction of all objective and subjective phenomena to some unknown physical stuff, the principle of physicalism rather implies a *methodological* reduction of the study of all natural phenomena to the theories and research methods of the physical sciences.

This brings us once again to the question: are the methods devised for the study of objective, physical phenomena sufficient for the scientific study of subjective, mental phenomena? At this point, all answers are expressions of faith, for it is obvious that physical and biological sciences have not yet comprehensively explained the origins, nature, or causal efficacy of consciousness or any other mental phenomenon. Great advances have been made recently in discovering the neural correlates of an increasing range of mental processes, but none of these explains the so-called "hard problem" of how these physical events give rise to subjective experience. Scientific materialists confidently declare that eventually, the time-tested methods of physics and biology will unravel the mystery of consciousness, fulfilling Antonio Damasio's hope of using the tools of neurobiology to comprehensively explain subjective experience in terms of neural patterns. But there are compelling reasons for skepticism about the neurobiological reduction of the mind to the brain.

Despite centuries of modern philosophical and scientific research into the nature of the mind, at present there is no technology that can detect the presence or absence of any kind of consciousness, for scientists do not even know what exactly is to be measured. Strictly speaking, *at present there is no objective, scientific evidence even for the existence of subjective experience!* All the direct evidence we have is based on introspection, but this mode of observation has yet to be developed into a rigorous means of scientific inquiry. The root of the problem is more than a temporary inadequacy of the technology. It is rather that modern science does not even have a theoretical framework within which to conduct experimental investigations.

Cognitive scientists commonly gauge the success of their research by the extent to which they are able to identify the "underlying mechanisms" of mental processes. This insistence on finding mechanical explanations was equally common among physicists until the late nineteenth century, when it was discovered that natural phenomena, such as electromagnetism, cannot always be understood in terms of mechanisms. The mature discipline of physics has learned this through hard experience. But younger branches of science, especially the cognitive sciences, whose models of neural function are generally based on nineteenth-century physics, are still captivated by the Cartesian belief that something is truly explained only if its underlying mechanisms have been identified. Physicists have long ago abandoned that ideal; cognitive scientists may eventually be forced by their own empirical research to do so as well.

Given the fact that contemporary physicists are so little concerned with the real, objective nature of matter, the ontological division between "material" and "immaterial" also needs to be readdressed. Since the late nineteenth century, physicists have operationally defined electromagnetic fields as oscillations of abstract field quantities in space. More broadly, many now view all configurations of mass-energy as oscillations of abstract field quantities in space. Given the conceptual nature of such quantities, the reified division between material and immaterial seems to melt away.

Proponents of scientific materialism draw a sharp distinction between the naturalism of science and the supernaturalism of religion. And naturalism, or the belief that all natural phenomena can be fully explained in terms of other natural phenomena, is equated with materialism. Advocates of supernaturalism, in contrast, insist that the world cannot be fully understood without acknowledging the role of a transcendent God who created and intervenes in the natural world. While this debate will undoubtedly continue for the foreseeable future, here I would simply like to challenge the notion that all natural phenomena must be material in nature.

Electromagnetic fields, the probability waves of quantum mechanics, the vacuum states of quantum electrodynamics, and the eleven dimensions of contemporary string theory can certainly be deemed natural. But how meaningful is it is classify them as "material"? Since physicists have jettisoned matter as some metaphysical stuff whose mechanisms account for all natural phenomena, it is time to consider alternatives to the naïve assumptions of both monistic materialism and Cartesian dualism. While the latter fails to explain how nonphysical mental processes could influence the brain, monistic materialism equally fails to explain how the brain produces subjective mental processes. Scientific materialism has limited scientific thinking to metaphysical categories rooted in the seventeenth century, and science itself has shown that these categories are outdated.

Implications for Education and Society at Large

Let us now consider the results of the fusion of science and scientific materialism in the American educational system. The way science is commonly being taught in public schools has failed to provide many students with a sound understanding of even its most rudimentary aspects. Surveys suggest that most people in the United States today can't tell an atom from a molecule from a cell, lack even a basic understanding of electromagnetism, don't know the difference between a star and a galaxy, and don't understand genetics or the outline of natural history on this planet. This is quite remarkable if we consider how much money and effort has been invested over the last forty years in public science education.

Scientific materialists such as Edward O. Wilson declare that science is bound to dispel all traditional religious beliefs, like one species wiping out another species that is competing for the same biological niche. But recent polls taken in the United States suggest that the empirical evidence may not support his claim. According to one, most Americans believe in ghosts, one third accept astrology, and one fourth believe in reincarnation.[18] A Gallup poll taken in 2000 found that 83 percent of Americans and 49 percent of Europeans feel God is very important in their lives.[19] If the encounter between science and religion is viewed as a battle between the mind and the heart, the heart appears to be winning. While in some regions of the United States, science, together with the assumptions of scientific materialism, is freely taught, in large parts of the country a heated backlash is taking place in public education against any scientific theories being taught that contradict a literal interpretation of the Bible. In such areas, the chasm between science and religion seems to be widening. But is such conflict necessary? For the sake of society as a whole, should we not explore how the two can coexist and perhaps even complement each other?

The twentieth century may rightly be called the century of scientific materialism, when this worldview came into its full strength. This was the greatest century in the history of humanity in terms of the growth of scientific knowledge, but the worst century in terms of man's inhumanity to man and the general degradation of our natural environment. The most murderous despots the world has seen, including Stalin, Hitler, and Mao Zedong, were able to enlist the services of scientists in perpetrating their crimes against humanity. And numerous scientists and engineers in the free world have applied their knowledge and ingenuity to developing weapons of mass destruction that now terrorize humanity as a whole. While many scientists have abided by high ethical standards, the metaphysical framework of scientific materialism gives them no incentive for doing so. Indeed, by reducing human subjectivity to neural processes occurring according to the impersonal laws of physics, it undermines any sense of moral responsibility.

Life, Liberty, and the Pursuit of Happiness

The 2004 national elections in the United States revealed an unprecedented degree of ideological and emotional polarization of the American public against itself and the rest of the world. The alienation between the warring factions was due in large part to the fact that each found the other's position incomprehensible. "How can anyone who loves God and country support Kerry?" was the challenge posed in churches and synagogues throughout the heartland of America, and "How can any reasonable, informed person who cares about the world as a whole support Bush?" was the rhetorical question posed in colleges and universities throughout the nation.

The polarization that characterizes the American public today focuses on familiar themes:

> reason vs. faith
> facts vs. values
> head vs. heart
> cities vs. rural areas
> cosmopolitan vs. parochial
> science vs. religion
> self-reliance vs. reliance on authority
> realism vs. idealism
> materialist values vs. spiritual values

George W. Bush thoroughly embodies one side of this divide, and the values he consistently represents and champions found widespread support when the nation was traumatized by the attacks of September 11, 2001. His policies have so uniformly advocated the second of all the above polarities that he has become a powerfully appealing symbol for those who lean to the Right, and a powerfully repulsive symbol for those who lean to the Left. As a result of this deeply antagonistic polarization, there is little room left in the middle, and hardly any ground for mediation between the two extremes. Many citizens who supported Bush in the 2004 election did so because of what he stands for in their eyes—especially his moral values—*despite what they perceived he had done over the preceding four years and planned to do during his second term.* Many swing voters, on the other hand, refused to vote for Kerry because he appeared to stand for so little, despite what he promised to do if elected president.

This polarization can only be understood in the historical context of Western civilization, which is rooted in two radically different cultures: the Greco-Roman and the Judeo-Christian. Many powerful thinkers, including Augustine, Aquinas, Galileo, Newton, and Kant, have sought to reconcile the worldviews, values, and ways of life promoted by these two cultures. But now their incompatibility has crystallized in the division within the American public and the alienation of much of the rest of the world.

This split began as a problem in the Mediterranean basin; it then became a European problem, then an American problem; and with the modern spread of the Euro-American worldview, values, and way of life, it has become a global problem. Militant, fundamentalist Muslims also cherish the latter of each of the above polarities; but unlike President Bush, they loathe the Euro-American worldview, values, and way of life, regarding them as antithetical to their own worldview, values, and way of life based on the Qur'an. One form of religious fundamentalism violently collides with another, despite their extensive common orientation and values.

The disparity between the Greco-Roman and Judeo-Christian heritages has become nothing short of a kind of social bipolar disorder, and in those who try to embrace both poles, it often results in a sort of "doublethink." Many devout Christians and Jews enthusiastically support scientific research and embrace the fruits of technology, yet have not come to terms with the fact that the physical sciences portray a universe that has no role for a personal God who intervenes in nature and responds to the prayers of the faithful. And they turn a blind eye to the fact that the biological sciences portray humans as physical organisms devoid of an immortal soul imbued with free will. Likewise, many advocates of scientific materialism are ethical people with a strong sense of social responsibility, but their own views support the materialistic attitude and rampant consumerism that are destroying our natural environment and undermining human values. While reducing human identity to brain functions operating under the control of the impersonal laws of physics and biology, they look in vain for any realistic basis for personal responsibility or ethics, let alone any spiritual dimension of human existence or the world at large.

The world is now in dire need of fresh, integrative perspectives to heal this existential fragmentation. They must include a mediating ideal of a meaningful life that draws on and honors both heritages while transcending their polarization. To seek this ideal, let's reappraise the vision of the American Founding Fathers when they sought to establish a nation that upheld the ideals of life, liberty, and the pursuit of happiness within the context of a meaningful life.

Life: Cherish the lives of all humans, regardless of nationality, ethnicity, or creed, and all sentient beings, human and nonhuman, including unborn embryos that are either human or in the process of becoming human, and the entire ecosphere, which is essential for the flourishing of life on our planet.

Liberty: Cherish the freedom of all peoples for self-determination and the exercise of their basic human rights. Seek freedom from the inner causes of misery and conflict, such as greed and self-centeredness, hatred and animosity, and ignorance and delusion.

The pursuit of happiness: Cherish the well-being of everyone. With discerning intelligence, draw from the religious heritages of humanity for guiding ethical principles, and let scientists examine what forms of behavior truly result in genuine happiness and flourishing for individuals and society as a whole. A central emphasis of such research should be eliminating poverty and starvation throughout the world. Likewise, let medical science continue to diagnose and treat illnesses, and ensure that everyone is provided with basic health care. Let the mental health sciences explore the nature not only of mental disease but also of mental health, including exceptional states of mental balance and well-being.

As noted in the preceding chapter, the pursuit of genuine happiness, or human flourishing, is an ancient ideal from our Greek and Christian heritage. Certainly such happiness, as opposed to mere transient pleasures, must be based on truth, but what kinds of truth? For Jews and Christians, this is fundamentally the truth of God and mankind's creation in the image of God. For Socrates it was self-knowledge. The religiously minded seek the truth from the top down by relying on the authority of divine revelation, while the scientifically minded seek the truth from the bottom up by relying on human empirical and rational inquiry. These two approaches have collided head-on, but is there any way they might turn out to be complementary? The greatest impediment to finding out is the presence of powerful elements of dogma in both religion and science. Religion has become largely a matter of belief and adherence to divinely decreed ethical standards, while science is dominated by the principles of materialism, which many of its advocates acknowledge are articles of faith, not empirically confirmed scientific facts.

Neither religion nor science alone can claim sole authority for understanding the nature of human identity or the world around us. The human mind cannot be thoroughly comprehended only through the scientific examination of the brain and behavior; the human soul cannot be fathomed only on the basis of divine revelation. Science is not equipped to explore the spiritual dimensions of existence, for its tools have been designed to measure physical processes. Science and religion may yet prove to be complementary, but only if adherents of both return to the primacy of experience.

The same principle holds true in terms of the cultivation of virtue, which Aristotle and Augustine both acknowledged to be indispensable for the pursuit of genuine happiness. But virtue must also be based on truth. Indeed, a life of virtue may be viewed as a life that reflects the nature of truth. Science has forgotten this principle, as it has become evident over time that one may become a great scientist—with great insights into certain aspects of reality—without cultivating virtue and without reaping the fruits of genuine happiness. But religion has also fallen into the error of ignoring the empirical insights of science in determining what kinds of behavior are truly conducive to human flourishing within the context of the individual, family, community, nation, international community, and entire ecosphere. Let a spirit of empiricism and critical inquiry prevail, and humanity may explore and embrace a revitalized sense of ethics and virtue that is both inspired by the religions of the world and empirically tested by the methods of science.

As global economies are fast depleting the nonrenewable, physical resources of our planet, there is now an urgent need to explore the inexhaustible, inner resources of the human spirit and to utilize them in the common pursuit of life, liberty, and the pursuit of happiness for all beings. In this way, the human civilization may find harmony within itself and in relation to the rest of the ecosphere.

SCIENTIFIC MATERIALISM AS A RELIGIOUS DOGMA

One way of determining whether an ideology conforms to the category of "religion" is to see whether it directly collides with religious dogmas. Imagine the following statements being made in the public school system by teachers who hold sectarian religious beliefs.

- A Jew states that Jesus was not the Son of God and the miracles attributed to him in the New Testament never occurred.
- A Hindu states that it is not true that there is but one God, Allah, and Muhammad is his prophet.
- A Buddhist states there is no divine creator who governs the universe.
- A Taoist states that the Jews are not God's chosen people and he did not enter a unique covenant with them.
- A Christian refutes the existence of reincarnation and karma.
- A Muslim refutes the possibility of achieving salvation by one's own efforts, without believing in God.

In the United States it is illegal to make any of the above assertions, *or their opposites*, in a public classroom even if the teachers in question do not promote the truth of the rest of their own religious beliefs or teach their creed as a unified whole. Advocates of scientific materialism, however, make all the above claims, explicitly or implicitly, in public classrooms *and* promote their own belief system as a coherent, integrated ideology. *The more the ideology of materialism is conflated with science in the public educational system, the more we can expect religious fundamentalists to insist that their ideologies are also taught in science classrooms.* In this way, the division between religion and science will broaden.

The split between church and state in the United States is based on the First Amendment to the Constitution, which says, "Congress shall make no law respecting an establishment of religion, or prohibiting the free exercise thereof." The original meaning of this amendment is that Congress shall not select and shall not establish any particular church in order to make it into what would be an American equivalent of the Church of England. The broader purpose was also clear: to prohibit Congress from having any negative impact on the free exercise of religion through governmental favoritism of one denomination over another, for example, by officially recognizing and subsidizing it as *the* national church.

But the current, widespread interpretation goes far beyond the original intent. On the basis of the First Amendment, the U.S. Supreme Court has repeatedly ruled against the teaching of religion in public schools, although the teaching of religious history, the philosophy of religion, sacred text as literature, and comparative religion is permitted. The scope of the amendment hinges upon the determination of what is and is not a religion.

In Edward O. Wilson's presentation of scientific materialism in his well-known book *Consilience*, he has a great deal to say about the realm of human purposes, meaning, and value, which is widely viewed as the proper domain of religion. Wilson also writes at length on our ultimate origins and destiny and the experiences of our inner life. In scientific materialism the boundaries between science and religion dissolve, and a new religion is presented as a substitute for all traditional religions. The sacred object of its reverence, awe, and devotion is not God or spiritual enlightenment but the material universe, which exists transcendently "outside our heads." In other words, scientific materialism appears to be a modern kind of nature religion, or neoanimism, which had innumerable precedents in the preliterate history of humanity. As such, it appears to be one giant step backward for mankind.

If we were to follow the original intent of the First Amendment, scientific materialists should be required, at the very least, to subject their claims to open, critical scrutiny. Since scientific materialism has been deemed "scientific" rather than "religious," a different standard has been applied to the promotion of its ideology. The restrictions of the First Amendment are not only evaded but also misinterpreted so that only one religious doctrine is promoted in the state educational system: scientific materialism. During the twentieth century, the U.S. government has interpreted the First Amendment in the spirit of the French revolution, which persecuted traditional religion in the name of a new "scientific religion." This is a far cry from the orientation of the American Revolution, which promoted freedom from governmental establishment of one state religion in favor of freedom for all religions.

Most religions are communal, having their own institutions and rituals, and scientific materialism is no exception. The vast majority of elite scientists—members of the National Academy of Sciences and tenured faculty at the most prestigious institutions of learning—are staunch scientific materialists.[20] So their institutions, including state universities, serve as the host institutions, or surrogate churches, for this faith. And in Marxist countries, where scientific materialism is the dominant worldview for society as a whole, governments have acted as institutions to promote and enforce this ideology. The brutality and intolerance that traditional religions have exhibited is well known, and many people have abandoned religion altogether for that reason alone. Unfortunately, the same tendencies have been expressed by the institutions of scientific materialists. This is most evident in communist countries, where members of other religions have been systematically persecuted, subjected to forceful conversion, torture, and mass murder due to their beliefs. In democratic nations, such brutal suppression of nonmaterialistic beliefs is not permitted, but more subtle pressures are commonly applied for students and faculty to conform to the dictates of scientific materialism.

While the ideologies of traditional religions and of scientific materialism differ in content, in many respects they are very much alike. As Wilson admits, the principles of scientific materialism "cannot be learned by pure logic; for the present only a leap of faith will take you from one to the other."[21] The validation of this leap of faith, he declares, will eventually be reached through the accumulation of objective evidence acquired by scientists, with biologists leading the way. Thus, the creed's ultimate validation rests on the authority of future biologists, who will take on the role of messiahs to redeem humanity from its present ignorance and delusion.

TEACHING RELIGION AND SCIENCE IN THE STATE EDUCATIONAL SYSTEM

Since the twentieth century, the First Amendment has been interpreted to mean that government-run schools in the United States are prohibited from teaching any religion as true, and they must on no account adopt any as the state religion. However, the world's religions have undeniably exerted a powerful and often ubiquitous influence on the development of human communities. To understand any society's internal functioning and relation to other societies, an understanding of its religious beliefs, practices, and institutions is indispensable.

Unfortunately, in American primary and secondary schools, education in the world's religions tends to be marginalized, often so overlooked that graduating high school students have little understanding of any of the world's religions unless they happen to have been brought up in a religious household. During the twentieth century, religious beliefs have been demoted to the status of mere opinions that may be deemed true if one simply believes in them enough.

In the latter half of the twentieth century, the academic field of religious studies in secular universities arose by defining itself in contrast to theology. Consequently, scholars of religion are required to assume a position of neutrality in regard to the material they are teaching. They must be seen to be floating above the subject matter, as it were, and alighting nowhere. This may well be embraced as a suitable pedagogical stance as long as it is equally applied to all types of religious beliefs, including those of scientific materialism. But in practice, the writings of Emile Durkheim, Marx, Freud, and other proponents of scientific materialism are commonly included among the required reading in classes on religion. Adoption of the principles of materialism and reductionism promoted by these detractors of religion is commonly viewed as an objective outlook, a proper educational methodology, whereas any traditional religious views are seen as subjective. And subjectivity is the central taboo of scientific materialism.[22] It should hardly come as a surprise then that many students who take courses in religious studies find their faith in religion devalued. They are brought under the sway of scientific materialism whether they take courses in science or religion!

In American public schools, science education is often conflated with scientific materialism, and this may be one reason students wind up learning so little about actual science. As noted previously, the majority of Americans, given their religious orientation, reject scientific materialism, so it is unlikely that the quality of education can be improved in the long run by identifying science with this worldview. Moreover, the worst kind of science education is the kind that tells students it is wrong to question the authority of any dogma. Sooner or later, students are bound to see the implications of scientific materialism, and in many cases this leads to an unfortunate disillusionment with science as a whole.

The way to shed light on the relation between science and religion is to encourage teachers, students, and researchers to explore the relationship between scientific knowledge and beliefs on the one hand, and religious knowledge and beliefs on the other, and to see where they overlap. This requires reintroducing a spirit of true empiricism into the study of both subjects, and that students are introduced to the ethical, historical, and philosophical contexts in which the sciences and religions of the world have emerged and coevolved throughout history. Science has the potential for providing a wonderful bridge for interreligious dialogue and for comparative religious studies, while helping to sharpen philosophical reflection and deepening our appreciation of these received wisdom traditions. William James writes in this regard,

> Let empiricism once become associated with religion, as hitherto, through some strange misunderstanding, it has been associated with irreligion, and I believe that a new era of religion as well as philosophy will be ready to begin....I fully believe that such an empiricism is a more natural ally than dialectics ever were, or can be, of the religious life.[23]

The current separation of science and religion is exaggerated by the conflation of empirically demonstrated facts and dogmatically held beliefs. In the spirit of the authors of the American Constitution, it is time to readdress what is meant by the establishment of religion and the free exercise thereof. As we identify the illusions of knowledge presented as fact in the dogmas of scientific materialism and the rest of the world's religions, we may open up new vistas of discovery that transcend the current borders between science and religion.

3

THE STUDY OF CONSCIOUSNESS, EAST AND WEST

THE ACHIEVEMENTS OF scientific inquiry fill us with wonder as researchers probe the inner core of atomic nuclei, galactic clusters billions of light-years away in space, and events during the first nanoseconds after the Big Bang, 13.8 billion years away in time. But for all its marvelous success in illuminating the objective world, from the extremely minute to the extremely vast and distant in space and time, science has kept us in the dark regarding the origins, nature, and potentials of our own subjective consciousness. Progress in understanding the natural world as a whole—including its objective and subjective aspects and the relation between them—has been radically lopsided. And this has created a skewed sense of human identity and the nature of the universe.

Why has Western civilization failed to develop a science of consciousness? It is not as if the nature of consciousness, which is crucial to human identity, has not been deemed important in the Western tradition. Socrates addressed this point: "I am still unable, as the Delphic inscription orders, to know myself; and it really seems to me ridiculous to look into other things before I have understood that."[1] Some propose that since consciousness is intrinsically such an elusive, mysterious phenomenon, it is only fitting that science should have taken so long before probing its nature. But immediate knowledge of our own consciousness is, arguably, our most certain knowledge, as Descartes proposed in his *Meditations*—more certain than our knowledge of the objective, external world. Moreover, it is only by way of consciousness that we have any sense of the rest of the world.

HISTORICAL IMPEDIMENTS TO THE EMERGENCE OF A SCIENCE OF CONSCIOUSNESS IN THE WEST

I turn first to the twin roots of Western civilization: the Greco-Roman and the Judeo-Christian traditions. One pivotal element in the emergence of a new science is the development and refinement of instruments to observe and experiment with the phenomena under investigation. Galileo's use of the telescope to examine the sun, moon, and planets played a crucial role in the emergence of the science of astronomy. Likewise, Van Leeuwenhoek's use of the microscope to observe minute life forms was crucial to the emergence of modern biology. It is therefore reasonable to assume that a science of consciousness should be heralded by the development and refinement of an instrument with which states of consciousness can be observed with rigor and precision. The only instrument humanity has ever had for directly observing the mind is the mind itself, so that is what must be refined.

Many Western scientists and philosophers have argued that the alleged introspective observation of mental events is radically unlike observation of celestial phenomena with a telescope. While the mind would ostensibly have to observe itself, the telescope is directed at something to which it bears only an external and contingent relationship. As philosopher John Searle comments, "Any introspection I have of my own conscious state is itself that conscious state ... the standard model of observation simply doesn't work for conscious subjectivity."[2] When introspection is characterized as "the mind observing itself," this suggests that a single, unified entity—the mind—is observing one thing—itself. But when we generate a mental image of a rose and observe it, this bears at least some similarity to observing the visual image of a rose. For most people, the mental image is far less stable, vivid, and detailed, but those who are even moderately adept at visualization can report at least on the color of the rose they are imagining. And while such an image is held in the mind, it does appear to be an *object* of attention, not the subjective awareness of that mental object.

To take another example, with even a little practice it is possible to detect discursive thoughts and images that arise and pass in the mind. Noting such thoughts is very much like overhearing phrases of a conversation held in another room, and witnessing such images is akin to observing appearances sporadically flashing on a television screen. Moreover, in a dream one observes a wide range of mental phenomena corresponding to the five physical senses, and there is a clear sense that the entity experiencing these events is not identical to the mental appearances themselves. This is all the more obvious in the case of a lucid dream, that is, when the dreamer clearly apprehends that he or she is dreaming.[3]

In short, experience shows that subjective awareness is not necessarily identical to the mental phenomena of which it is aware, any more than it is identical to the sensory images of physical phenomena by which we apprehend the world around us. The mind observing itself is not like a telescope being directed at itself. It is more like a system of measurement detecting quantum mechanical events that are distinct from but related to the measuring device. Both are instances of "observer participation." When we observe a thought or note that we are experiencing a certain emotion or desire, this immediately influences the detected phenomenon. This obviously does not happen when observing planets with a telescope. But this type of interaction between the system of measurement and the measured phenomena is characteristic of quantum mechanics. So there is no reason to believe that the phenomena to be studied scientifically must invariably exist independently from the means of observation.

In his refutation of introspection (while at the same time, quixotically maintaining that the first-person perspective on mental phenomena is primary), Searle argues, "The idea that there might be a special method of investigating consciousness, namely 'introspection,' which is supposed to be a kind of inner observation, was doomed to failure from the start, and it is not surprising that introspective psychology proved bankrupt."[4] There are far more compelling reasons the primitive methods of introspective psychology in the West were unsuccessful, the most important of which is that the quality of attention applied to the task was inadequate.

Untrained attention is habitually prone to alternating bouts of agitation and dullness, so if the mind is to be used as a reliable tool for exploring and experimenting with states of consciousness, these dysfunctional traits need to be replaced with stability and vividness. While the philosophers of ancient Greece were certainly interested in the nature of the mind, there is little evidence that they developed any sophisticated means for refining the attention. The Pythagorean brotherhood and the mystery schools may have devised such methods, but if they did, specific knowledge has not been preserved. Jewish mystics also wrote extensively on the nature of consciousness,[5] but the development of techniques to cultivate attentional stability and focus for the rigorous exploration of consciousness was not a strong suit of their tradition either.

Within the Christian tradition, the early desert fathers were certainly aware of the need to calm the mind, as is evidenced in the seminal fifth-century volume on contemplative practice entitled *The Conferences of Cassian*.[6] But it is not clear how effective Christian contemplatives of that period or the later medieval era were in devising methods for training the attention in order to observe mental events. The widespread conclusion among Christian mystics that the highest states of contemplation are necessarily fleeting, commonly lasting no longer than about half an hour, may indicate the limitations of their attention training.[7] This insistence on the ephemeral nature of mystical union appears to originate with Augustine,[8] and it is reflected almost a millennium later in the writings of Meister Eckhart, who emphasized that the state of contemplative rapture is invariably transient, with even its residual effects lasting no longer than three days.[9]

The advent of the Protestant Reformation and the scientific revolution hastened the decline of Christian contemplative inquiry into the nature of consciousness. Given the Protestant emphasis on the Augustinian theme of the essential iniquity of the human soul and man's utter inability to achieve salvation or know God except by faith, there was no longer any theological incentive for such inquiry. Salvation was emphatically presented as an undeserved gift from the Creator. So genuine happiness, which is to be truly experienced only in the hereafter, is in no way earned by understanding the mind or achieving exceptional states of mental health and balance.

René Descartes and John Locke were both deeply committed to the introspective examination of the mind, but like their Greek and Christian predecessors, they did not devise means to refine the attention so that the mind could reliably be used to observe mental events. Moreover, Descartes declared that the soul is divinely infused into the body, where it exerts its influence by way of the pineal gland. He believed that this gland induces the voluntary actions of the body, while all other actions are reflexive. This belief may account in part for the fact that the scientific study of the mind did not even begin for more than two centuries after his time. The mind was deemed to be outside the scope of the natural sciences, which were focused on the external, objective world of matter. Indeed, until the last three decades of the nineteenth century, the pineal gland was uniquely neglected by physiological and biochemical investigators. Although various factors may be responsible for this scientific avoidance, it seems plausible that one reason was that that region of the brain was still considered to be outside the proper domain of natural science.

Another trend in Europe at the dawn of the modern era provided yet a further incentive for not delving deeply into the human mind: the witch-hunting craze from the late fifteenth century through the mid-seventeenth century. During this period, anyone who exhibited exceptional mental powers, including the power of spiritual healing, was immediately suspected of being a witch. Nearly all traditional societies have believed in witchcraft, but the Christian tradition in particular attributed the powers of witches to the devil, which is the rationale for the biblical commandment that such people are to be put to death.[10] The common belief that demons and other spiritual entities roved about in the natural world (sometimes taking possession of human souls) was deeply incompatible with the emerging mechanical view of the universe. After all, scientists couldn't very well establish orderly physical laws in the objective world as long as there were immaterial spirits at large, intervening at will in the affairs of man and nature. So many natural philosophers of the late sixteenth century simply dismissed them as illusions. But there was still a widespread belief that the human soul was vulnerable to demonic possession, which could be seen as a warning sign to beware of the depths of the human mind. It was another two hundred years before psychoanalysts had the nerve to begin the scientific exploration of this dark inner wilderness.

In short, the trajectory of Western science from the time of Copernicus to the present seems to have been influenced by medieval Christian cosmology, according to which hell was symbolized as being in the center of the earth and heaven as in the outermost reaches of space. Likewise, especially according to the dominant theology of the Protestant Reformation, the soul of man, at the subjective center of human experience, was a den of iniquity, and the only chance for salvation was to look to a source of good absolutely *outside* the human mind. In this light, it hardly seems an accident that the discipline that initiated the scientific revolution was astronomy—studying the phenomena most distant from the perceiving subject—and that the scientific discipline of psychology took a full three hundred years to develop. And only in the closing years of the twentieth century did the scientific community begin to regard consciousness as a legitimate subject of scientific inquiry.

Although various psychologists, including William James, were interested in consciousness in the nineteenth century, by the early twentieth century, the topic had become taboo, particularly in American academia. This was due in large part to the fifty-year domination of academic psychology by behaviorism. In 1913, the American behaviorist John B. Watson, as mentioned previously, declared that psychologists must avoid the use of all subjective terms such as "sensation," "perception," "image," "desire," "purpose," and even "thinking" and "emotion" as they are subjectively defined. And he attributed belief in the very existence of consciousness to ancient superstitions and magic.[11] Forty years later, B. F. Skinner echoed this theme by asserting that mind as such does not exist at all, only dispositions for behavior. Another decade elapsed before the futility of equating subjective mental processes with objective behavioral dispositions became apparent to the scientific community. The behaviorist approach did nothing to explain the nature of the mind, let alone consciousness; it just reduced these subjective phenomena to a class of objective processes that could be studied with the available tools of science.

With the emergence of cognitive psychology during the 1960s, subjective experience was once again allowed back into the realm of scientific research, but the role of introspection in exploring the mind was still marginalized, just as it is in the rapidly progressing field of neuroscience. Rather than equating mental processes with behavioral dispositions, cognitive psychologists and neuroscientists now equate them with neural processes and their functions. Cognitive neuroscientists have discovered many types of causal relationships between the mind and the brain. They have found that mental processes are disrupted in various ways when the corresponding brain activity is disrupted, and that a wide range of cognitive processes influence neural activity. Such discoveries essentially boil down to the following correlations: specific neural events (N) are correlated to specific mental events (M), such that if N occurs, M occurs; if M occurs, N occurs; if N doesn't occur, M doesn't occur; and if M doesn't occur, N doesn't occur. Such correlations could imply that the occurrence of N has a *causal* role in the production of M, or vice versa; or it could imply that N and M are actually the same phenomenon viewed from different perspectives. There is not enough scientific knowledge at this point to determine which is correct. Moreover, while the dualist hypothesis leaves unexplained how immaterial, subjective mental events could possibly influence the brain, the materialist hypothesis leaves equally unexplained what enables the brain to produce conscious experience of any sort. There are unresolved, hard problems on both sides of this fence, but materialists seem much more convinced about the difficulty of explaining how consciousness emerges from matter.

Mental events viewed introspectively appear to be radically different types of processes than neural events viewed objectively. Moreover, exclusive focus on the introspective examination of the mind reveals little if anything about the brain. *If brain scientists were to confine their research to the brain alone, without reference to any first-person reports of mental experience, they would not learn much about the mind. Indeed, they would have no reason, on the basis of neural events alone, to conclude that they are correlated to any mental events at all.* Some neuroscientists account for this lack by acknowledging that they know relatively little about the brain, in contrast to knowledge of the mind acquired through centuries of introspection.[12] But biologist Edward O. Wilson, on the contrary, maintains that logic launched from introspection is limited and usually unreliable, which is why even today people know more about their automobiles than they do about their own minds.[13] The consensus among psychologists is that introspection is an unreliable means for investigating the mind. As for our current understanding of the mind and consciousness, Daniel Dennett and John Searle comment, respectively, "Consciousness stands alone today as a topic that often leaves even the most sophisticated thinkers tongue-tied and confused,"[14] and "Where the mind is concerned we are characteristically confused and in disagreement."[15]

If scientists were presented with a new instrument for observing a specific type of natural phenomenon, the first logical step to take before using it would be to examine its nature, including its strengths and limitations. Does this instrument merely present its own artifacts, like looking into a kaleidoscope does, or does it provide data that exist independently? If the instrument does yield such objective information, does it distort it or provide objective data? Only after they had understood the design, functioning, reliability, and capacities of the instrument could they confidently use it to collect data.

The primary instrument that all scientists have used to make every type of observation is the human mind. Does this instrument provide only its own artifacts, without access to any objective reality existing independently? If the mind provides information about the objective world, does it distort it in the process? For reasons outlined above, the scientific study of the mind in the West was delayed for three centuries after the scientific revolution; this is tantamount to using an instrument for three hundred years before subjecting it to scientific scrutiny.

Wilson, as seen previously, expresses the view of many scientists when he asserts that outside our heads is an independent, objective world, and inside our heads is a reconstitution of reality based on sensory input and the self-assembly of concepts. The proper task of scientists, he claims, is to correctly align our inner representations of reality with the world outside.[16] The problem here, which he acknowledges, is that scientists have no body of external, objective truth by which the alignment of scientific theories and the world outside can be calibrated. In other words, the empirical data that we perceive, together with the scientific theories that account for them, all consist of mental representations; and we have no objective yardstick with which to compare them with what we assume to be the "real world."

How are we to get out of this conundrum? Wilson suggests that "criteria of objective truth might be attainable through empirical investigation. The key lies in clarifying the still poorly understood operations composing the mind and in improving the piecemeal approach science has taken to its material properties."[17] He assumes that the mind is actually composed of brain processes, but as I have already pointed out, this is still an unproven hypothesis, not a scientifically established fact. Given how little scientists presently understand about the relation between the mind and the brain, it would be far more objective to regard it as a topic to be researched with an open mind, rather than assuming (or demanding) that science will one day confirm current materialistic beliefs.

If we maintain this materialistic bias, no empirical science of consciousness is likely to emerge in the foreseeable future. Rather, if the cognitive sciences continue to be constrained by the assumptions of scientific materialism, consciousness will be reduced to something that *can* be explored and understood within the parameters of that ideology, as various researchers, such as Francis Crick and Christof Koch, are already attempting to do.[18] Just as kinematics (the phenomenological study of matter in motion) logically precedes mechanics in the study of physics, the rigorous, firsthand investigation of consciousness logically precedes any formulation of the mechanisms that account for the emergence of consciousness.

Modern science has never developed a rigorous introspective methodology for observing the phenomena of conscious mental processes and states. William James, the foremost pioneer of American psychology, recognized the importance of studying behavioral and neural correlates to mental processes, but he emphasized the primary role of introspection in this endeavor.[19] However, insofar as the mind is prone to alternating agitation and dullness, it is an unreliable instrument for observing anything. To transform it into a suitable instrument for scientific exploration, the stability and vividness of the attention must be developed to a high degree. James was well aware of the importance of developing such sustained, voluntary attention,[20] but he acknowledged that he did not know how to achieve this task.[21]

To sum up, the modern West has developed a sophisticated science of behavioral and neural *correlates* of consciousness, but no science of consciousness itself, for it has failed to develop sophisticated, rigorous means of exploring the mental phenomena firsthand. And that is the first step toward developing an empirical science of *any* class of natural phenomena. Thus, with regard to exploring the nature, origins, and potentials of consciousness, cognitive scientists and neuroscientists are more like astrologers, who carefully examine *correlates* between celestial and terrestrial phenomena, than astronomers, who carefully examine celestial phenomena themselves.

A second result of the historical development of Western science is an elaborate science of mental illness, but no science of mental health. Indeed, there is hardly any scientific consensus on the criteria by which to identify mental health. Nor is there any Western science that shows how to cultivate extraordinary mental health or genuine happiness. The Greek and Christian theories of *eudaimonia*, the human good and a "truth-given joy," have been forgotten in modern science,[22] and the very existence of a truth that yields such well-being has no place in the scientific view of human existence or the universe at large.

In short, the West presently has no *pure* science of consciousness that reveals the nature, origins, and potentials of this natural phenomenon, and it similarly lacks an *applied* science of consciousness that reveals means for refining and enhancing consciousness and thereby achieving *eudaimonia*. But this does not necessarily imply that all other human civilizations throughout history have been equally deficient.

THE BUDDHIST SCIENCE OF CONSCIOUSNESS

Over the course of its 2,500-year history, Buddhism has developed rigorous methods for refining the attention, and then applying it to explore the origins, nature, and role of consciousness in the natural world. The empirical and rational investigations and discoveries by such great Indian contemplatives as Gautama Buddha profoundly challenge many assumptions of the modern West, particularly those of scientific materialism. The interface between Buddhist and modern Western science also challenges our very notion of "metaphysics." In the nineteenth century, the origins of the physical universe, the constitution of distant galaxies, and the internal structure of molecules were all matters of philosophical speculation. There were no known ways of exploring these topics empirically, but that is no longer the case. In the twenty-first century, the nature, origins, and destiny of human consciousness are still philosophical issues for the West, but they are not similarly shrouded in mystery within the Buddhist tradition.

As new empirical strategies are devised for exploring phenomena, speculation is supplanted by knowledge. Buddhist contemplatives have always placed a primary emphasis on fathoming the nature of the mind, and their orientation to this endeavor has been fundamentally pragmatic. In general, the framework of Buddhist theory and practice consists of the Four Noble Truths: the truths of suffering, the source of suffering, the cessation of suffering together with its source, and the path leading to that cessation. The first task in Buddhist practice is to recognize the nature and full range of suffering to which humans are vulnerable. The second noble truth presents the hypothesis that the essential causes of suffering are to be found as imbalances within the mind. The third noble truth hypothesizes that these afflictive tendencies can be irreversibly dispelled from the mind. And the fourth noble truth presents an integrated path of ethical discipline, the development of *samādhi* (including all aspects of mental balance), and contemplative inquiry into the nature of the mind and other phenomena as means for transforming the mind and eliminating its afflictions and obscurations.[23]

In Buddhist contemplative practice, the experiential investigation of the mind, including the nature, origins, and potentials of consciousness, is of paramount significance. But in order for such exploration to be penetrating and reliable and for the insights gleaned to be thoroughly assimilated, the attentional imbalances of laxity and excitation must first be eradicated. Only when the attention is lucid and calm can it be used effectively in this venture.[24] This point is brought out in an eighth-century Indian Buddhist meditation classic called *Stages of Meditation*:

> Because the mind moves like a river, it does not remain stationary without the foundation of quiescence. The mind that is not established in equipoise is incapable of knowing reality. The Lord, too, declared, "The mind that is established in equipoise discovers reality."[25]

The Tibetan Buddhist contemplative and philosopher Tsongkhapa (1357–1419) wrote in a similar vein:

> When examining a tapestry in a dark room, if you illuminate it with a radiant, steady lamp, you can vividly examine the images. If the lamp is dim, or, though bright, flickers in the wind, your observation will be impaired. Likewise, when analyzing the nature of any phenomenon, support penetrating intelligence with unwavering, sustained, voluntary attention, and you can clearly observe the real nature of the phenomenon under investigation.[26]

According to Buddhist tradition, the qualities of luminosity and stillness are innate to the substrate consciousness, so the central challenge of this training is to settle the attention in that ground state. One of the remarkable discoveries of Buddhist contemplatives who have penetrated to this stratum of consciousness is that it is imbued with an innate quality of bliss. In other words, when the attention is settled in this deep state of equilibrium, temporarily free of laxity and excitation, one experiences a sense of inner peace and well-being. To reach this dimension of consciousness, a necessary prerequisite is the cultivation of a wholesome way of life that supports mental balance and harmonious relations with others. This is the essence of Buddhist ethics, which is the foundation of all Buddhist practice.[27]

Simply settling the attention with a high degree of attentional stability and clarity is not enough to irreversibly free the mind of its afflictions and obscurations. This requires penetrating to the level of primordial consciousness, transcending the conceptual demarcations of subject and object, mind and matter, and even existence and nonexistence. Such consciousness is metaphorically described as being empty and luminous, and never sullied by afflictive imbalances of any kind. Its realization is said to yield a state of well-being beyond imagining, and this represents the culmination of the Buddhist pursuit of freedom from suffering by way of knowing reality. With such insight, it is said that one comes to understand not only the nature of consciousness but also its relation to the world of experience. *Insight into the deepest dimension of consciousness is therefore the key to understanding the nature of reality as a whole.*

With this understanding of three dimensions of consciousness—beginning with the psyche, extending to the substrate consciousness, and culminating in primordial consciousness—the Buddhist view of the mind challenges many common assumptions in the modern West. According to many psychologists today, the normal mind is healthy, but is nevertheless subject to various kinds of mental distress, including depression, anxiety, and frustration. When these problems become excessive, they are treated with drug therapy and counseling. While unhappiness, it is said, comes simply from being human, happiness seems to come from outside: from sensual and aesthetic enjoyments, from possessions, from relations with other people, and, according to religious believers, from God. The Western view of the mind is still influenced by the Aristotelian assertion that all emotions, in the appropriate circumstances and in moderation, are to be accepted.[28] This belief has been incorporated into the theory of evolution, and some evolutionists maintain that all our emotions and other mental traits must have facilitated our survival and procreation, otherwise we wouldn't have them.

In contrast to the above views, Buddhist contemplatives state that the ordinary mind is dysfunctional, for it is prone to all kinds of imbalances, including the attentional problems of succumbing to the turbulence of involuntary thoughts and emotions and slipping into dullness. We have grown habituated to experiencing such a dysfunctional mind and mistakenly take for granted the resultant mental discomfort, believing this to be normal and acceptably healthy. So we take solace in outer and inner pleasurable stimuli, which suppress the dysfunctional symptoms. While the normal mind is *habitually* prone to states of conative, attentional, cognitive, and affective imbalances, it is not *intrinsically* dysfunctional. By refining the attention, we can make the mind serviceable and thereby discover the innate sense of well-being that emerges spontaneously from a balanced mind. And by fathoming the nature of primordial consciousness, all the obscurations of the mind may be removed, resulting in freedom from suffering and its source.

TOWARD AN INTEGRATION OF BUDDHIST AND WESTERN SCIENCE

While the scientific study of consciousness has achieved legitimacy in recent years, it is overwhelmingly dominated by the assumptions of scientific materialism. The influence of this belief system does little to impede progress in the physical sciences, but it has a constricting effect on the biological sciences (including medical science) and even more so on the cognitive sciences. One of its most limiting aspects is that it places a taboo on the empirical investigation of subjective events from a first-person perspective. And there is a widespread refusal among researchers in this field even to consider the possibility that mental events may be immaterial in nature, not simply epiphenomena or functions of the brain.

If Buddhist tradition has indeed developed a science of consciousness, why is this not commonly acknowledged? On the one hand, it emphasizes an introspective approach to the study of the mind, the value of which is not commonly accepted among scientists. But there are other compelling reasons. Over the centuries Buddhism has repeatedly fallen into dogmatism and scholasticism, while marginalizing its original emphasis on empiricism and pragmatism.[29] The trend of regarding the Buddhist teachings simply as a body of belief has been exacerbated by much modern academic scholarship in the field of Buddhist studies, which lends little credence to the exceptional experiences and insights of Buddhist adepts, refusing even to consider the possibility that they may have made extraordinary discoveries pertinent to our contemporary understanding of the mind and its role in nature. In the most extreme cases, Western Buddhologists[30] go so far as to claim that experience has never played a prominent role in Buddhist practice. But the problem is not just in the *representation* of Buddhist practice in the West. Over the centuries, the spirit of open-minded inquiry has faded among many Buddhist scholars and contemplatives. This has gone so far, according to one contemporary Tibetan Buddhist scholar, that the primary concern of many Buddhist meditators is mainly to ensure that they are following the correct procedure of a meditation technique, rather than rigorously exploring the nature of the mind or anything else.[31]

During the Renaissance, Europe emerged from the shackles of religious dogma in part because of the influx of fresh and provocative ideas from classical Greece and the Arab world. Now the West, and all other countries dominated by it, is in need of a renaissance to free it from the intellectual tyranny of scientific materialism, which is often conflated with science itself. The Buddhist tradition, especially if it is reinstilled with the spirit of empiricism and skepticism, may play an important role.

Researchers of the mind-body problem commonly appeal to the authority of future scientists to confirm their present materialistic assumptions about the nature of consciousness. Antonio R. Damasio, for example, claims, "It is probably safe to say that by 2050 sufficient knowledge of biological phenomena will have wiped out the traditional dualistic separations of body/brain, body/mind and brain/mind."[32] It took the scientific community fifty years to recognize that the mind couldn't meaningfully be reduced to a set of behavioral dispositions. Now many cognitive scientists are committed to explaining all mental phenomena solely in terms of neural activity. Once again, due to an ideological bias, the first-person experience of mental phenomena is marginalized or neglected.

While science characteristically embraces the "disturbingly new," it has a much harder time embracing the "disturbingly old," namely, discoveries that were made long ago (let alone in an alien civilization), prior to the scientific revolution. Many Buddhists, on the other hand, rely so heavily on the insights of the Buddha and succeeding scholars and contemplatives of the past that they have a hard time embracing disturbing new discoveries that challenge Buddhist beliefs. Scientific materialists are so confident that the mind is nothing more than a biological phenomenon that they confuse this belief with scientific knowledge. Similarly, many traditional Buddhists are so confident of the validity of their doctrines that they confuse their belief with contemplative knowledge. Daniel J. Boorstin comments that the great discoverers of the past "had to battle against the current 'facts' and dogmas of the learned."[33] This battle must now be waged on at least two fronts: the scientific and the religious.

The scientific tradition is beginning to join the Buddhist tradition in its pursuit of understanding the nature, origins, and potentials of consciousness. At this point in history, neither on its own embodies a rigorous, unbiased, multifaceted science of consciousness that includes the detailed, integrated study of the broadest range of mental phenomena and their neural correlates. Buddhism embodies a wealth of insight drawn from the first-person exploration of normal to exceptional states of consciousness, but it has little to say about mental disease, the psychological effects of brain damage, or the neural correlates of mental phenomena. The cognitive sciences have yet to develop rigorous methodologies for the first-person study of the mind, and since they have largely confined themselves to studying the behavioral and neural correlates of normal and subnormal minds, they leave us in the dark about the higher potentials of consciousness.

Without the use of the telescope, medieval astrologers would never have discovered the moons of Jupiter, spots on the sun, or craters on the moon—let alone the myriad astronomical discoveries since the time of Galileo—regardless of the care with which they examined the terrestrial correlates of celestial phenomena. Likewise, without developing heightened degrees of attentional stability and vividness, as is done in Buddhist meditative practices, cognitive scientists have little chance of discovering a wide range of mental phenomena that have allegedly been ascertained by accomplished contemplatives in the past. Among the experiential discoveries claimed by Buddhist contemplatives are the continuity of individual consciousness beyond death, reincarnation, the possibility of achieving a wide range of paranormal abilities and modes of extrasensory perception, and the possibility of freeing the mind of all its afflictive tendencies. No reasonable Buddhist would ask scientists to accept any of these claims merely on faith—the Buddha himself discouraged his followers from accepting his words simply on the basis of his own authority—but it is equally dogmatic to dismiss them simply because they violate the principles of scientific materialism.

The value of collaboration between Buddhist contemplatives and scientists in terms of enriching our scientific understanding of consciousness may be evident, but the potential benefits for Buddhism may be less clear. After all, the point of Buddhist practice is to purify the mind of its afflictions and obscurations and thereby achieve a lasting state of well-being. By its own accounts, it has done this quite successfully without knowledge of the brain. So what possible advantages could such collaboration hold for the Buddhist tradition?

Over the past 2,500 years, Buddhism has traveled to and become assimilated in a variety of civilizations throughout Asia. Throughout this long history, it has maintained theoretical acuity and practical utility by engaging with the host societies *at the highest levels of theoretical discourse and experiential inquiry.* If it is to sustain such relevance in today's world, it cannot afford to turn its back on the cognitive sciences, which are exploring many of the aspects of the mind that have long been of central interest in Buddhism. Moreover, while many Buddhist contemplative practices have proven their efficacy for exploring and transforming the mind in the traditional societies of Asia, these are now being introduced in the modern West, where circumstances are very different. Buddhist practices have always been adapted to specific people, times, and places, so they are inevitably being adapted in today's world as well. Among the hundreds of meditation techniques taught by the Buddha and later Buddhist adepts, which are most effective for people today? Are some more effective for certain types of people than for others? In what ways might they be adapted for optimal benefits?

These are pressing questions for Buddhists who are concerned with maintaining the vitality of their own tradition, and the cognitive sciences may be of great assistance in providing answers. In developing attention skills, for instance, behavioral and neurophysiological studies may help to reveal which techniques are most effective for inducing stability and vividness. The methods of the empirical sciences may also help illuminate which types of Buddhist practices are most effective in developing conative, cognitive, and affective balance. There have already been too many cases of Western meditators diligently practicing meditation ineffectively or even to their own detriment. So it makes sense to draw on all our current resources to maximize the benefits of such practices. As scientists and contemplatives collaborate in the investigation of the mind, which is so central to human existence, perhaps a comprehensive, fully integrated science of consciousness may emerge to the benefit of both traditions and the world at large.

4

SPIRITUAL AWAKENING
AND OBJECTIVE KNOWLEDGE

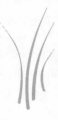

TWO IDEALS OF OBJECTIVITY

I will begin this discussion with an overview of the Buddhist ideal of objectivity, citing a well-known verse from the treatise *Four Hundred Stanzas* by the Indian Buddhist scholar and contemplative Āryadeva (170–270 C.E.):[1]

A suitable listener is said to be one who is
Objective, intelligent, and earnest.
Such a one will not misconstrue the qualities
Of either the speaker or the listener.

A "suitable listener" is an individual fit to follow the Buddhist path to spiritual awakening. Such a person must be objective in the sense of being unbiased, not demonstrating an irrational preference for their own views or an aversion to the views of others. In addition, a suitable trainee for the Buddhist path must be intelligent in terms of knowing how to distinguish between robust and defective theories, and be earnest in a respectful and attentive way, engaging with Buddhist teachings with the aspiration to put them into practice. One should ideally be free of not only personal but also cultural biases, which may be much harder to identify. A cultural bias is a dominant culture's superimposition of characteristics, attitudes, or abilities on the basis of stereotypic assumptions about the "true nature" or "proper role" of a given nondominant cultural group. It is therefore the result of an inclination, or a preconceived opinion or predisposition, to decide a cause or an issue influenced by any consideration other than its merit.[2] Such cultural bias often masquerades as a healthy sense of skepticism, which is necessary in both Buddhism and science, but it shows its true face when that skepticism is directed only toward the assumptions of others and not of oneself or one's own culture.

In the Buddhist pursuit of liberation (*nirvāṇa*) and spiritual awakening (*bodhi*), strong emphasis is also placed on freeing oneself from the contaminating influences of mundane concerns, including the classic, eightfold list of material gain and loss, stimulus-driven pleasure and pain, praise and ridicule, and peer acceptance and rejection. Moreover, in the course of Buddhist practice, one is encouraged to examine what attitudes and emotions are conducive over the long run for achieving the ideal of freedom through insight. Finally, the Buddhist ideal of objectivity entails transcending the limitations of ordinary human consciousness and exploring reality with a mode of awareness that is beyond all subjective human concepts and language. The primary strategy for pursuing this ideal is the cultivation of *samādhi*, based upon a prior training in ethics and followed by the investigation of phenomena with this refined mode of mental perception.[3] The underlying assertion is that humans *internally* have access to states of awareness that transcend the subjective limitations of the mind as such.[4]

The scientific ideal of objectivity, originally expressed as the pursuit of a "God's-eye view," is deeply rooted in Christian theology. A common belief among Christian theologians during the era of the scientific revolution was that those who seek wisdom and eternal intellectual life receive it only by a gift of grace. Wisdom thus originates from an absolutely *objective* source, namely God, and people become receptive to it insofar as they are freed from all *subjective* human influences. In this theology, the human self is depicted as "a wretched sinner" and "a paltry creature" who bears "a corrupt nature"[5]—all of which are very good reasons to be free from any kind of subjective influence! The strategy for those seeking the divine life and eternal wisdom, according to this theological stance, is adopting a virtuous life, observing the commandments, showing outward devotion, mortifying the flesh, and cultivating contempt for the mundane things of the world. Any emphasis on cultivating focused attention, as in Buddhist contemplative practice, is conspicuously absent.

This goal of achieving a God's-eye view of nature was explicitly adopted by Galileo and many other pioneers of the scientific revolution, who turned their attention *outward* in their pursuit of objective truth. Many of them envisioned that this would culminate in a kind of *apotheosis*, when man's understanding of the natural world would merge with the understanding of God.[6] It is important to recognize, though, that from early on, the scientific ideal of objectivity has involved more than freedom from human conceptual biases. Rather, the quest has been to penetrate beyond the "veils of appearances" of the human senses and beyond the limitations of human concepts and languages. Technological advances in the development of many data-gathering devices and systems of measurement have facilitated the ideal of distancing the human senses from scientific empirical inquiry. And with the use of mathematics, Galileo and other early "natural philosophers" believed that they could objectively think in God's own language.[7] But modern science has never devised means to refine the attention so that introspection can be rigorously used to explore the mind and its relation to the rest of reality.

During the latter half of the nineteenth century and especially throughout the secularizing trend of the twentieth century, the traditional pursuit of a God's-eye view came to be supplanted by the pursuit of what has been called "a view from nowhere."[8] The fundamental ideal remains the same: the perspective of a disengaged observer, capable of objectifying the surrounding world and suppressing emotions, inclinations, fears, and compulsions in order to pursue research in an unbiased and rational manner. This implies a taboo against subjectivity, which refers to all conscious and unconscious personal influences, including individual consciousness itself and all personal, individual goals, attitudes, and points of view. Subjective experiences are thus described in the objective terms of the natural sciences, and the physical world is assumed to be purely objective. The inevitable result of this exclusion of subjective experience is that scientific knowledge of reality is viewed as something entirely separate and independent from issues such as the meaning of life, the pursuit of happiness, the cultivation of virtue, human values, and ethics. Given the above criteria for objective research, it is unreasonable to expect to discover meaning, which is intimately related to subjective awareness, in the universe as portrayed by science. If meaning is to be discovered, either it will have to be found by nonscientific means or science will have to expand its modes of empirical research.

THE SCIENTIFIC PURSUIT OF OBJECTIVE KNOWLEDGE

The scientific pursuit of objective knowledge of nature has traditionally been based on the absolute Cartesian distinction between the objective, material world and the subjective, immaterial mind. This prescientific, metaphysical position places both the human mind and the mind of God outside of nature, and hence outside the domain of natural science. Where do all our sense impressions of the physical world, such as the appearances of colors, fit into this bifurcation of reality? Edward O. Wilson addresses this point explicitly: "Color does not exist in nature. At least, it does not exist in nature in the form we think we see. Visible light consists of continuously varying wavelength, with no intrinsic color in it."[9] According to Descartes, color is but one of many secondary attributes—including sounds, smells, tastes, heat, cold, and other tactile sensations—that exist only in relation to sense faculties. They do not exist objectively in the real, outer world. Nevertheless, Wilson, in line with the writings of many neurophysiologists, goes on about the recognition of color *in the brain*,[10] without explaining—or even addressing—how the experienced appearance somehow arises. After all, when we look at a red rose, no brain cells actually turn red; when we taste wine, our brain cells don't taste like wine; and when we smell a rose, its fragrance is not to be found in the brain. Yet all these qualities, according to Descartes, are not located in the world outside either. The implication is that all our sensory impressions of the objective world exist nowhere in the objective world, neither outside nor inside the brain!

This peculiarity does not seem to perturb many scientists, for science is primarily concerned with exploring the objective world existing outside and independently of all sensory impressions. As noted previously, modern science relies heavily on technological instruments for detecting physical phenomena, and on the basis of the appearances, or data, produced by such instruments, scientists devise ingenious models and theories to explain the objective processes that give rise to those phenomena. It should immediately be obvious that such data result from both the objective processes in nature and the specific kinds of measuring devices used to detect them. They do not exist independently in nature any more than experienced colors or sounds do.

This problem is particularly salient in the field of quantum mechanics, in which light, for example, displays wave properties when detected with one type of measurement system and particle properties when detected with another. This problem is further compounded by the fact that, in some as yet inexplicable manner, unmeasured quantum processes exist only as potentialities, but as soon as they are measured, they become realities. As discussed previously, the very nature of matter, as a kind of objective, locally existent, independent stuff, becomes more and more problematic the more deeply one probes into the nature of the physical universe. Some physicists are now speculating that *information*, rather than *matter*, may be the fundamental stuff of nature.[11] But just as it is awkward, if not impossible, to posit the existence of real quantum processes independently of any system of measurement, it is at least as problematic to posit the existence of information independently of any cognitive system, such as a human mind. Information that does not inform is not information at all. And for the act of informing to take place, there must be a conscious agent to receive the data.

One of the central principles of modern physics is the conservation of mass-energy. But if information is an even more fundamental constituent of the universe, one can legitimately ask whether there is a similar conservation principle for it. Freud concluded that "In mental life nothing which has once been formed can perish ... everything is somehow preserved and ... in suitable circumstances ... it can once more be brought to light."[12] As soon as the mind is returned to nature, from which Descartes unnaturally removed it, conservation principles can be seen at work in terms of objective mass-energy, subject-object-related information, and subjective mental events. Following this line of inquiry, as physicist Erwin Schrödinger surmised,[13] the barriers between subject and object begin to break down. Or one begins to recognize that such absolute barriers never exist outside the realm of imagination.

The scientific exploration of the mind and its relation to physics has been a long time coming, especially since it was not even initiated until roughly three hundred years after the scientific revolution. There were good reasons for this delay. As noted previously, Descartes and like-minded individuals excluded the mind from nature; and over the next three centuries, the instruments of science were designed to explore objective, not subjective phenomena. And in principle there is something fundamentally problematic about trying to objectively explore a range of phenomena that is, as philosopher John Searle cogently argues,[14] irreducibly subjective. Edward Wilson suggests that the exclusion of human mental life from natural science "turned out to be a healthy decision for the profession of science, because it steered researchers away from the pitfalls of metaphysics."[15] But Wilson's sanguine diagnosis of this lack of parity between the scientific study of objective and subjective phenomena assumes that the exploration of the mind inevitably leads to "the pitfalls of metaphysics." There seems to be no reason in principle why the mind should be any more mysterious than the origins of the universe or the structure of quarks, which are considered to be very much part of physics, not metaphysics, by cosmologists and particle physicists. The real issue seems to be whether or not scientists can devise empirical means

of exploring the nature of mental phenomena, not just their neural and behavioral correlates.

The mind is supremely important for testing the metaphysical axioms of
scientific materialism, for, as Wilson points out, "Everything that we know
and can ever know about existence is created there."[16] Many contemporary
scientists would have us skip the first step of developing precise means to
explore the subjective appearances of mental phenomena. In short, contrary
to the development of physics, they would like to go straight to the objective mechanisms in the brain that are correlated to mental phenomena. As
Wilson argues, "The fundamental explanation of mind is an empirical rather
than a philosophical or religious quest. It requires a journey into the brain's
interior darkness with preconceptions left behind."[17] Although he claims that
this approach is empirical, in fact it marginalizes mental processes as they
are experienced firsthand. And while he promotes the ideal of leaving behind
preconceptions in this pursuit of understanding, this method is itself satu-
rated with the metaphysical preconceptions of scientific materialism, which
he never seriously questions. One of these, of course, is his assumption that
cellular events actually compose the mind, which has yet to be demonstrated
in any neuroscientific laboratory.

Firsthand observation of mental phenomena has not always been marginalized in the history of psychology. Primitive forms of introspection were
used extensively during the closing decades of the nineteenth century, but
the data derived from such observation were found to be untrustworthy. And
instead of refining the mind so that introspection could be made into a more
rigorous method, psychological research has largely excluded introspection
ever since—for reasons both pragmatic and metaphysical.[18] Where science
has made extraordinary progress, especially during the past few decades, is in
the study of brain functions and their relations to specific mental processes.
But as Wilson acknowledges, contemporary neuroscience cannot yet explain
how patterns of neuronal firing create the full scenarios of consciousness.[19]
Neuroscientists and philosophers of mind commonly join in the assertion
that consciousness somehow emerged over the course of evolution and occurs in the development of a human fetus due to the complex interactions of
large numbers of cells. But since they do not know the precise nature of the
complexity required to produce consciousness, this hypothesis has no real
explanatory or predictive power. In fact, it fails every test of a truly scientific
theory and must therefore be deemed a metaphysical assumption. And the
fact that modern science has no objective means of detecting the presence or

absence of consciousness in anything provides little hope that the assumption can be scientifically tested anytime in the foreseeable future.

The Cartesian notion that reality fundamentally consists of two kinds of entities—mind and matter—has largely fallen into disrepute in both scientific and philosophical circles. One reason is that this dualistic model was never able to explain how a nonphysical mind could influence physical phenomena. But it is easy to turn the tables on this argument: the monistic model of matter being the only real stuff in the universe has never explained how the matter in the brain, for instance, gives rise to mental phenomena. Nor does it explain how mental attitudes, beliefs, hopes, intentions, desires, and the like exert influence on the body, both as voluntary actions and as "placebo effects." A common basis of both Cartesian dualism and materialist monism is their assertion of the real, objective existence of matter, as opposed to mind. But such matter exists, according to Immanuel Kant, in a noumenal realm that is finally unknowable *in principle*. Kant was no more optimistic about understanding the real nature of the mind, independent of all appearances. An empirical science of the mind, he declared, is impossible, for the true basis of mental phenomena is as inaccessible to inner experience as the true basis of physical phenomena is to outer experience.[20] But in Kant's reification of both the knowable, phenomenal worlds of mental and physical realities and the unknowable, noumenal world, there is no explanation of how the phenomenal and the noumenal can ever interact. A common basis among the metaphysics of Cartesian dualism, materialist monism, and Kantian idealism is the belief in real, independent entities. And it is in this assertion that the scientific pursuit of objective knowledge fundamentally diverges from the Middle Way (Madhyamaka) view of Buddhism.

THE BUDDHIST PURSUIT OF OBJECTIVE KNOWLEDGE

It is questionable whether scientific research has truly unveiled the nature of a purely objective reality existing independently of all appearances and conceptual frameworks. But it has certainly been enormously successful in revealing innumerable truths about the natural world of phenomena perceived *within the context of conceptual frameworks*. The early records of the Buddha's discourses have a term for this world of experience—*loka*—and this, not some purely objective universe allegedly existing independently of experience, is the focus of the Buddhist pursuit of knowledge.[21] The Buddha added, however, that the world we experience as human beings is not the only world; there are others in addition to our own. But all these worlds are said to be "unreal" and insubstantial, like a bubble or a mirage.[22] Later Buddhists have interpreted these characterizations of phenomena in various ways, but a common theme is that there is an incongruity between the way things appear and the way they actually exist. This, of course, is also a central theme of science.

There are, nevertheless, many significant differences between scientific and Buddhist pursuits of objective knowledge, in terms of methods and goals. According to Galileo and the majority of the founders of modern science, salvation is granted by an act of divine mercy, which one receives by faith, by surrendering to the will of God, and by applying oneself to a life of virtue in accordance with God's commandments. This is the way to achieve meaning and goodness in this life and salvation in the hereafter. The practice of science, in contrast, entails an intellectual challenge to understand the objective, physical universe. This not only is unnecessary for salvation but also can be pursued independently of any concern for meaning, virtue, or heavenly rewards. Nevertheless, some of the pioneers of the scientific revolution, such as Francis Bacon, believed that the development of experimental science was sanctioned by God as a means for understanding and controlling nature. Thus, faith was seen as the key to inner happiness, and scientific knowledge was seen as the key to material well-being. This split between the goals of science and religion is every bit as radical and far-reaching in its implications as Descartes's absolute demarcation between mind and matter.

When he left the comforts of his home and family at the age of twenty-nine, Gautama—the Buddha-to-be—set out to "seek what is good," which, he envisioned, would lead to "the supreme state of sublime peace." But he chose a path primarily involving the pursuit of knowledge, as opposed to the adoption of faith in the hope of divine rewards. His first step was to seek out the most accomplished contemplatives of his day to learn from them how to refine his own mind. The first of his teachers, Āḷāra Kālāma, initially gave him practical instructions on a range of increasingly subtle states of meditative concentration. Gautama surmised that he was not simply speculating on these matters but was reporting direct knowledge from his own experience, and when he questioned him on this matter, Āḷāra Kālāma confirmed that this was indeed the case. According to early Buddhist accounts, Gautama then engaged in a meditative discipline under the guidance of his teacher. In a remarkably brief time he achieved Āḷāra Kālāma's own state of focused attention, in which the mind gains access to a formless dimension of existence that is devoid of all content apart from an experience of pure nothingness. His teacher was so impressed at his extraordinary progress that he invited Gautama to teach with him, but Gautama felt that this state alone did not fulfill his deepest aspiration. He then sought out an even more accomplished contemplative named Uddaka Rāmaputta, under whose guidance he achieved an even subtler state of meditative absorption that transcended the very concepts of discernment and nondiscernment.

In both these meditative states, the mind transcends the world of sensory experience and even the realm of mental imagery, and for as long as one remains in such a state, one remains profoundly at peace. But Gautama recognized that meditative absorption alone did not reveal the true nature of reality or result in "the supreme state of sublime peace." Moreover, after one emerges from such meditation and engages with the everyday world, the mind is still prone to suffering and its underlying causes. Gautama seems to have taken very much to heart the principle that only truth can make one free, and it is evident from the beginning of his spiritual venture that he was not satisfied merely to accept others' theories on the basis of authority and tradition.[23]

As indicated by Gautama's initial meditative training, Indian contemplatives of his day had apparently learned how to refine and focus the attention in extraordinary ways, far surpassing anything known to modern science. It was on the shoulders of these contemplative giants that he developed his own unique methods for using the mind to explore the nature of reality. In the earliest records of Gautama's own narration of his achievement of spiritual awakening, he describes how, with his mind concentrated, purified, malleable, and calm, he recollected the specific circumstances of many thousands of his own former lives over the course of many ages of world contraction and expansion. This, he declared, was his "first true knowledge" on the night of his awakening, gained through his own direct experience. He next proceeded to observe the succession of lifetimes of other beings, ascertaining the relations between their deeds and their effects as they played out in subsequent lives. He reported, "I understood how beings pass on according to their actions. This was the second true knowledge attained by me in the second watch of the night."[24] Finally, his contemplative insight into the nature of reality was so thorough that his mind was utterly freed from all afflictions and obscurations. This was his culminating realization of the Four Noble Truths: "I had direct knowledge, as it actually is, that 'This is suffering,' that 'This is the origin of suffering,' that 'This is the cessation of suffering,' and that 'This is the way leading to the cessation of suffering.'"[25]

It was at this point that Gautama became a buddha, "an awakened one," and he later reported:[26]

> When liberated, there came the knowledge: "It is liberated." I had direct knowledge: "Birth is exhausted, the holy life has been lived out, what was to be done is done, there is no more of this to come." This was the third true knowledge attained by me in the third watch of the night. Ignorance was banished and true knowledge arose, darkness was banished and light arose, as happens in one who is diligent, ardent and self-controlled.

The liberation that Gautama sought and found was freedom from *duḥkha*, our fundamental vulnerability to mental afflictions and suffering in this and in all possible future lives. The achievement of *nirvāṇa*, or spiritual liberation, brings with it the experience of a genuine, lasting state of well-being, or *sukha*, which stems from insight into the ultimate nature of reality. Contrary to all stimulus-driven pleasures, realization of such *sukha* arises from the very nature of pure awareness itself, freed from all afflictions and obscurations. It can be described as a state of human flourishing that is compassionately attentive to the joys and sorrows of others, is free of all tendencies toward vices such as malice and greed, and effortlessly gives rise to all virtues.

In the West, religion is often affiliated with transcendentalism, while science is associated with empiricism. This dichotomy is based on the premise that all empirical data are gathered through the five physical senses and the instruments of technology, which refine and extend those senses. In this context, the mind is commonly characterized as being comprised of representations of sensory impressions and the memory and imagination of them. The possibility of humans being endowed with a sixth mode of perception, namely mental perception, is rarely considered, let alone developed and refined. But it should be obvious that we are *directly aware* of our thoughts, emotions, desires, dreams, ideas, and mental imagery, and of the very existence of our own consciousness. We also mentally, not only sensorially, perceive our bodies and external environment. While the eyes perceive only visual objects and the ears perceive only sounds, with the mind we are capable of perceiving all manner of inner and outer phenomena, from the realm of mathematics to distant stars and galaxies. Perhaps our most robust, certain knowledge is the immediate knowledge of our own consciousness—something undetectable with all the instruments of modern technology. That which uniquely provides direct knowledge of mental phenomena is mental perception (*manas-pratyakṣa*), and Buddhist contemplative practice begins with the refinement and extension of this basic mode of observation.

As soon as mental perception is added to our faculties for observing reality, the scope of empiricism must include the full range of subjective mental events, which are so often excluded or marginalized in scientific research. In this regard, Buddhism, like science, can be said to be primarily an empirical, not a philosophical or metaphysical approach to understanding reality. There is an obvious complementarity between Buddhist and scientific empiricism. Buddhists meditatively refine and extend mental perception through the cultivation of mindfulness and introspection,[27] primarily as a means of exploring and controlling the mind. Scientists technologically refine and extend their physical senses as a means of exploring and controlling physical phenomena. As a result of such technological advances, scientists now have the use of a wide range of "extrasensory" modes of perception, such as radar, sonar, electron microscopes, and the like. Buddhist contemplatives claim to have developed a wide range of "extrasensory" modes of perception, such as remote viewing, precognition, and recollection of past lives.

Such claims quite rightly meet with skepticism from the scientific community. Given the current scientific understanding of the mind, it is hard to imagine how such modes of perception could be possible in principle. And given the lack of rigorous, scientific corroboration, it is hard for many people to take these claims seriously. But the history of science reveals that great leaps of progress have been made when the orthodox rules of scientific research have been broken. It does not seem impossible then, and certainly not undesirable, for science to expand its modes of empirical observation to include the refinement of mental perception and then put these Buddhist claims to the empirical test.

In Buddhist contemplative practice, after a sustained, rigorous training in developing the stability and vividness of attention, one then uses enhanced powers of mental perception to learn to distinguish between the phenomena that are presented to the senses and the conceptual superimpositions one compulsively imputes upon them. This entails the cultivation of discerning mindfulness[28] of the nature of the body, feelings, mental states, and all other outer and inner mental objects, examining, for instance, whether they are enduring or momentary, of the nature of *duḥkha* or *sukha*, and inherently personal or impersonal. Buddhist contemplatives, like scientists, are centrally concerned with all manner of causal relationships in the natural world. The Four Noble Truths, which provide the structure for Buddhist practice as a whole, are all about causality, with the central theme being the true causes of *duḥkha* and *sukha*. In this way, the Buddhist pursuit of knowledge is none other than the pursuit of the life of perfection and the realization of genuine happiness.

PERCEPTUAL KNOWLEDGE OF EVIDENT PHENOMENA

As noted in the previous account of Gautama's initial training with Āḷāra Kālāma and Uddaka Rāmaputta, from the very origins of Buddhism there has been a strong emphasis on the primacy of experience, or "direct knowledge," over conceptual inference, metaphysical speculation, or simple belief. This is reflected in the common response by the disciples of the Buddha to others who expressed an interest in his teachings: "Come and see!" (*ehi passi*). This emphasis entailed rigorous training in ethics and attentional training, which can reasonably be viewed as experiments in altering one's lifestyle and modes of attention. Buddhist contemplatives were then trained in using their finely honed attention to observe and analyze a wide range of inner and outer phenomena. If a mode of inquiry is deemed empirical if it is based on experiment and observation rather than theory alone, then Buddhist "insight" (*vipaśyanā*) meditation can be regarded as highly empirical. However, a major difference between Buddhist, contemplative empiricism and scientific, technological empiricism is that the latter involves quantitative measurements and sophisticated mathematical analysis, resulting in the formulation of precise mathematical laws of nature. Buddhist empiricism, in contrast, is qualitative rather than quantitative, and it is primarily concerned with understanding and transforming conscious experience, rather than understanding and controlling the objective world that exists independently of it.

The theme of direct experience (Pāli: *paccakkhañāṇa*) is of central importance in early Buddhist literature,[29] and "experience" (*anubhāva*) and "direct perception" (*pratyakṣa*) are also key terms in later Indian Buddhist writings on meditation and epistemology. Nevertheless, the importance of experiential knowledge in Buddhism has recently been called into question by a number of Buddhologists, many of whom take a postmodernist approach to this field of study. Stephen Batchelor, for example, has declared that the Buddha did not even claim to have insights into the nature of reality based on his own contemplative experience.[30] Robert Sharf, pointing out that there is no premodern Japanese or Chinese lexical equivalent for "experience,"[31] claims that the importance of experience was first introduced into Buddhism by a handful of twentieth-century Asian religious leaders and apologists.[32]

Batchelor's claim is easily discredited by the above account of the Buddha's enlightenment, as well as innumerable other early narratives of the Buddha's life and teachings. Sharf's assertion is just as easily invalidated by the obvious presence of various terms denoting direct experience in Pāli, Sanskrit and Tibetan Buddhist literature. But Sharf's larger claim cannot so readily be dismissed as an indication of poor scholarship. One of his central premises is that the authority of prominent Buddhist commentators, such as Kamalaśīla, Buddhaghosa, and Chih-I, lay not in their access to exceptional states of experiential contemplative insight but in their mastery of and rigorous adherence to sacred scripture.[33] In a similar vein, upon finding no conclusive evidence that the fifth-century Indian Buddhist writer Vasubandhu was inspired by meditative experiences to adopt an idealist philosophical viewpoint within Buddhism, Johannes Bronkhorst concludes that this move was purely theoretical in nature—despite the absence of any conclusive evidence to that effect. However, in Tibetan Buddhism there emerged an important genre of "songs of meditative experience" (Tib. *nyams mgur*), such as *The Hundred Thousand Songs of Milarepa*, spontaneously composed by an eleventh-century contemplative, which are cited widely by Tibetan Buddhist scholars and contemplatives alike.[34] Moreover, within Tibetan Buddhism, the mode of meditative instruction that is traditionally most highly valorized is called "experiential guidance" (Tib. *myong khrid*), in which the mentor teaches his students from his own contemplative experience, not just from his theoretical training. This long-standing emphasis on experience is easily overlooked by scholars who have had no personal interaction with such accomplished contemplatives.

Sharf suggests that Buddhist meditation was never intended to result in the attainment of extraordinary states of consciousness, but was rather designed to eliminate mental defilements, accumulate merit, and achieve supernatural powers.[35] This is certainly true for a wide range of meditations within Buddhism, in which the real or imagined benefits were valued more than any experiences one might have while meditating. But this must not obscure the fact that experiential insights, especially those derived through "yogic perception" (*yogapratyakṣa*), are viewed as the most effective ways to purify the mind, accumulate merit, and tap the potentials of consciousness. Certain Buddhist scriptures and treatises have been deemed doctrinally authoritative based on the assertion that they themselves are either directly or indirectly based on authoritative contemplative experiences.

Buddhist tradition in India, Tibet, and other Asian countries has traditionally valued three ideals for Buddhist adepts: the scholar (*paṇḍit*), the contemplative (*yogin*), and the saint (*bodhisattva*). One may achieve greatness in any of these three ways without being especially adept at the other two, but the highest ideal within Mahāyāna Buddhism is to achieve excellence in all three. The eleventh-century Buddhist adepts Nāḍapāda (Naropa) and Atīśa, both of whom exerted a profound influence on Tibetan Buddhism, are traditionally presented as individuals who embodied all three ideals. Within the modern academic study of Buddhology, only the ideal of scholarship is valued, while Western Buddhists who strive to achieve either contemplative insights or saintly qualities are at times even ridiculed by academics.[36] As Sharf acknowledges, "Scholars of religion are not presented with experiences that stand in need of interpretation but rather with texts, narratives, performances, and so forth."[37] Thus, Buddhologists' refusal to engage in rigorous, firsthand, or even secondhand exploration of the types of experiences derived through Buddhist practice leads to a rationalistic and dogmatic approach to the study of the relation between Buddhist theory and practice. Empiricism is dismissed as a central theme in Buddhism largely because it is so lacking in academic Buddhist studies.

Even if one grants the importance of experience in Buddhist practice, one may still argue that this should not be called "empirical." As Buddhologist Luis Gómez rightly points out, the scientific use of this term includes methods of hypothesis testing and falsification, uncertainty and probability, and mathematical laws and predictability, all of which are alien to Buddhism.[38] Robert Sharf goes a step further in declaring that because of its ambiguous epistemological status and essentially indeterminate nature, personal experience, no matter how extraordinary, can never serve as a reference point for truth claims.[39] He concludes:[40]

> Thus, while experience—construed as that which is "immediately present"—may indeed be both irrefutable and indubitable, we must remember that whatever epistemological certainty experience may offer is gained only at the expense of any possible discursive meaning or significance. To put it another way, all attempts to signify "inner experience" are destined to remain "well-meaning squirms that get us nowhere."

This is a serious charge, and if it were true, it would undermine any constructive collaboration that would relate Buddhist contemplative experiences with empirical scientific findings. However, it would equally imply that the experiences of wine connoisseurs could never be reference points for claims about the quality of specific wines, and that there could not be any discursive meaning or significance to their experiences. Moreover, the experience of solving a mathematical proof and of all other types of mental phenomena—from internal chitchat to emotions to dreams—would also fall outside the realm of discursive meaning. But the notion that none of these experiences can be a reference point for truth claims is implausible, and it is no less unreasonable to assume that meditative experiences are uniquely immune to public discourse and the possibility of acting as the basis of truth claims.

While some contemplative experiences or realizations are said to be ineffable, many can be described to others, especially to those who engage in similar practices. For example, a group of meditators who devote themselves to sustained, rigorous training of focused attention are able to communicate many of their experiences with one another in ways that might be relatively unintelligible to people who have never meditated. The same holds true for scientific observations and discoveries. While some are hard to convey to nonscientists, all of them can be described and explained to fellow scientists, especially to those working in the same field of research. In the final analysis, *all* scientific observations boil down to multiple individuals' firsthand experiences, and when those experiences are similar—or *intersubjective*—they are regarded as third-person scientific observations. Just as epistemological certainty grows in proportion to this process of communal verification in science and mathematics, so it does in contemplative practice.

As I have argued elsewhere at considerable length,[41] mental phenomena can be observed and experimented on just as much as physical phenomena. To be sure, such contemplative, introspective empiricism must, due to its subject matter, differ significantly from scientific, extraspective empiricism, and the standards of rigor must accordingly differ between these two complementary modes of inquiry. Moreover, as William James pointed out more than a century ago, it is crucial to discard the Cartesian notion of introspective knowledge as being irrefutable and indubitable. Errors can be made while observing mental phenomena, just as they can while observing physical phenomena. Rigorous contemplative empiricism calls for the need to refine and extend mental perception, analogous to the scientific refinement and extension of sensory perception.[42]

How might one intersubjectively test or challenge the validity of meditative experiences? Traditionally, Buddhism has relied heavily upon "second-person" monitoring and evaluation of a student's meditative experiences by an accomplished mentor. This is the nature of a "guru-disciple" relationship, and it is in principle similar to the mentoring that takes place in a wide range of other fields of inquiry. However, according to Buddhist tradition, the mentor not only evaluates the student's verbal reports and behavior but also, optimally, has extrasensory access to the student's mind. Atīśa, for example, strongly emphasized the importance of achieving such clairvoyance, through the cultivation of *samādhi*, as an indispensable means for achieving spiritual awakening and serving the needs of others.[43] He seems to have taken for granted the possibility of this achievement, for in his writings he simply argues for its importance, without justifying that it can be done. The only way to test this claim scientifically is to engage in the modes of attentional training taught in Buddhism (or study those who do so) and see if they produce the effects claimed by accomplished Buddhist meditators. This would be an empirical, as opposed to a dogmatic, response to such an unorthodox truth claim.

The problem of evaluating truth claims based on meditative experience is largely the same as that of evaluating introspective reports in general, and in his classic work *The Principles of Psychology* William James proposed a threefold strategy for addressing this challenge.[44] The first part is the intersubjective evaluation of first-person reports of introspective experience; the second is the study of behavior associated with such internal experiences; and the third involves neuroscientific research into the brain correlates of such experiences. Traditionally, Buddhist contemplatives have employed only the first two means of evaluation, allegedly augmented by clairvoyant insight into others' mind states. In the modern study of comparative mysticism, the behavioral effects of contemplative insights are often overlooked. But in Buddhism, the achievement of advanced states of *samādhi* and contemplative insights are said to bring about observable transformations in outer behavior, accessible to public scrutiny. Rigorous scientific study of the neural correlates of meditative experiences is not a part of Buddhist tradition, but this also holds much promise for revealing important information about the nature of the state and trait shifts that take place due to sustained meditative practice.

Despite the great importance of both sensory and mental perception in Buddhism, it is also widely recognized that there is nothing irrefutable or indubitable about the truth claims based on such immediate experience. The seventh-century Buddhist epistemologist Dharmakīrti described four bases for perceptual error: 1) a defect in a sensory organ; 2) an objective basis for error, as in the case of perceiving the illusion of a circle when observing a quickly turning firebrand; 3) a locational basis for error, as in the case of seeing trees moving from a moving ship; and 4) misperception due to distortions in one's own mental state.[45]

Errors in observation and measurement are also common in empirical scientific research, and rigorous criteria are devised for distinguishing between genuine data and artifacts of the system of measurement. How does the Buddhist tradition determine the existence of something on the basis of valid cognition? Tsongkhapa offers the following three requirements:[46]

> Something is accepted to be conventionally existent if it fulfills the following criteria: (1) it is widely accepted in terms of conventional valid cognition; (2) it is not invalidated by another conventional valid cognition; and (3) it is not invalidated by suitable, analytical inquiry into its true nature, that is, whether or not it is inherently existent. If it does not fulfill those criteria, it is asserted to be nonexistent.

When Tsongkhapa refers to a "conventional valid cognition" (Tib. *tha snyad pa'i tshad ma*), he means not merely knowledge of conventional language usage. Rather, he is referring to modes of perceptual and inferential knowledge that engage with phenomena as they appear, without analyzing whether they exist by their own inherent natures, independent of the conceptual frameworks within which they are identified. In effect, he is stating that something can be deemed conventionally existent (i.e., existent within the context of a consensual conceptual framework) by means of a valid cognition, only in relation to another conventional valid cognition. This implies that no conventional valid cognition by itself can be regarded as an absolute, for further investigation may later prove it to be defective. Moreover, his third criterion states that nothing can be accepted as inherently existent—that is, existing by its own intrinsic nature, independently of all conceptual and verbal designations—if the absence of such existence is determined by another valid cognition.

The circular nature of these three criteria of existence and of valid cognition is readily apparent. Whether or not a given cognition is deemed valid, and whether or not an object of cognition is deemed existent, is determined by *internal criteria, with no recourse to any independent, objective reality.* Moreover, as Buddhologist Georges Dreyfus has well argued, both epistemic and pragmatic criteria have commonly been applied in judging these issues.[47] Buddhist meditation is fundamentally concerned with two themes: transforming the mind and using it to explore itself and other phenomena. For instance, a wide range of meditations are designed to refine the attention, attenuate destructive emotions, enhance wholesome emotions, and give rise to a greater sense of well-being. The effectiveness of those procedures is open to investigation with the tools of psychology and the neurosciences. Other meditations are designed to yield insight into the fundamental nature of awareness itself. Even though such insights may be ineffable, Buddhist contemplatives claim that they result in psychological and behavioral changes, and these may be subjected to scientific investigation.

The internal nature of testing the reliability of empirical data by both epistemic and pragmatic means is also characteristic of scientific inquiry. While early natural philosophers such as Newton were intent on discovering absolute truths about the natural world, scientists learned the hard way to take a more modest stance regarding their best observations and theories. They now aim to devise theories that give an intelligible account of the empirical phenomena known to contemporary science.[48] A good theory is one that provides a high degree of predictability and allows for the possibility of greater manipulation of and control over observed phenomena. The very idea of absolute certainty of any scientific knowledge is now widely regarded as a myth, but this has in no way diminished scientists' enthusiasm for making new discoveries, even though they may eventually be invalidated by later "valid cognitions."

It must be emphasized here that the great majority of discoveries made by Buddhist contemplatives are not of the ineffable, inconceivable kind that is said to be typical of mystical experience. This fact allows for a broad spectrum of meaningful discourse among experienced contemplatives, even though the discourse may be unintelligible to those who lack such meditative training and experience. But a similar situation holds true for all scientific research: "third-person" corroboration of experimental findings always refers to people who are professionally trained in the relevant area of research, not to the general public.

A final, and seemingly radical, distinction may be made between the domains of inquiry of scientists and Buddhist contemplatives. While scientists study the natural world, which lies within the domain of empirical observation, Buddhism is often portrayed as being concerned with the unobservable domain of metaphysics. By developing better and better ways of refining and extending modes of extraspective observation of the physical world through the development of technology, science has pushed back the border of metaphysics in terms of very small phenomena and phenomena that are distant in time and space. But we in the modern West have commonly assumed that the limitations of introspective observation of mental events are absolute and, as a culture, we have done virtually nothing to refine or extend our modes of introspective observation. Buddhist contemplatives, on the contrary, claim that those limitations are not absolute and that mental perception can be developed in extraordinary and unexpected ways. This implies that there may be domains of reality that are metaphysical for science, but not metaphysical (in the sense of nonexperiential or nonobservational) for Buddhism. And of course, the reverse appears to be true as well. The question of what is empirical and what is metaphysical, therefore, seems to be embedded in the perceptual capabilities of individual communities and individuals. The demarcation between these two domains is therefore relative, not absolute.

INFERENTIAL KNOWLEDGE OF HIDDEN OBJECTS

Like many Indologists before him, Johannes Bronkhorst has cogently argued that a tradition of rational inquiry developed in ancient India, in which Buddhism played a seminal and enduring role. According to his definition, a tradition of rational inquiry includes a system of rational debate, linked to systematic attempts to make sense of the world and our place in it. This primarily involves free and uninhibited discussion of all issues, even in areas that might encroach upon other sources of authority, such as tradition, revelation, or insight.[49]

At the dawn of the modern era in Europe, secular philosophy and science best exemplified such a tradition, and they arose in defiance of allegiance to the authority of the Bible and the medieval scholastic tradition. Over the past century, however, Western philosophy and science have been largely dominated by the ideology of scientific materialism. As I have argued elsewhere,[50] this has inhibited the spirit of open, rational inquiry in both disciplines. Bronkhorst identifies the Buddha as one of the earliest proponents of rational inquiry in India, and this is exemplified in his counsel to the inhabitants of the town of Kesaputta in the Indian kingdom of Kosala. These people expressed to him a high degree of skepticism regarding the many conflicting teachings of self-proclaimed authorities who had visited their village. In response, the Buddha encouraged them to be skeptical of all such doctrines, including his own. He then counseled them not to rely upon anecdotal evidence, tradition, the authority of religious texts, speculative opinions, merely plausible theories, or personal allegiance to charismatic teachers, and cautioned them against depending upon mere logic or appearances alone. Rather, on a highly pragmatic note, he advised them to identify for themselves what is wholesome and what is unwholesome—what truly leads to their own and others' well-being and what does not—and to follow that.[51]

Another expression of rational inquiry attributed to the Buddha declares: "Monks, just as the wise accept gold after testing it by heating, cutting, and rubbing it, so are my words to be accepted after examining them, but not out of respect [for me]."[52] Just as dogmatism often replaces critical inquiry in modern philosophy and science, so has it repeatedly influenced Buddhist thought at various times and places over the past 2,500 years. But this does not imply that a tradition of rational inquiry has never existed in Buddhism, only that this ideal is often stifled by ideology.

Although Indologists have long been trying to persuade Western philosophers of the existence of genuine philosophy in India, its omission in most Western academic departments of philosophy shows they have made little progress. Perhaps the reason is that Indian Buddhist philosophy, for instance, differs significantly from Western philosophy in ways that are hard to comprehend. Specifically, like science, Buddhist theories allegedly stem from exceptional modes of observing and experimenting with reality; they ideally lead to yet more penetrating ways of experiencing reality; and this interaction between theory and meditation yields pragmatic benefits for the individual practitioner as well as the surrounding society. In these ways Buddhism is unlike Western philosophy, for it contains some prominent elements that are more like science and others that accord with religion.

While the role of experience, or direct perception, is fundamental to Buddhism, logic and inference are also important, especially concerning phenomena that are hidden from direct perception. Buddhist logicians thus differentiate between evident (pratyakṣa) and hidden (parokṣa) objects. The former are accessible to direct perception, while the latter are not but are accessible to objective inference (vastubalapravṛttānumāna). This distinction is not based on the inherent qualities of the objects in question but is relative to the present capacity of specific perceivers. For example, fire is perceptible when it is in plain sight, but hidden from an individual perceptual perspective when it occurs behind a hill. In such a case, the presence of the hidden object of fire is logically inferred on the basis of its resultant smoke. In order to make this inference, one must be certain that the dark cloud billowing up from behind a ridge is indeed smoke, not, for example, a cloud of dust stirred up from dredging an open coal pit. Second, one must be certain that smoke can be produced only from fire, not from any other source.

According to classical Indian Buddhist logic, in order to causally infer the presence of fire on the basis of smoke, there must be a prior perception of fire producing smoke and the knowledge that smoke can be produced only in this way.[53] If fire had never been perceived—or if it were imperceptible in principle—its presence could not be conclusively inferred on the basis of smoke. This point raises some interesting problems in the domain of scientific inference. For example, the planet Neptune was first detected, but misperceived, by Galileo in 1612, and as late as 1830 it was still misidentified by John Herschel as a star. Its eventual discovery was based on mathematical analysis of the deviation of Uranus from its predicted orbit. That is, the result of the deviation in the orbit of Uranus was causally attributed to the presence of another, unseen planet. It is possible in principle that this deviation could have been caused by some other influence, so the mathematical inference alone was not entirely compelling. William James points out that any number of hypotheses may be considered by way of conceptual analyses, but the terminus of thought must be direct perception. Only then is the "virtual" knowledge of conceptual analysis alone retroactively validated.[54] This is precisely what happened in 1846, when Neptune was for the first time correctly identified through a telescope.

The scientific problem of causal inference is considerably more problematic, however, when the objects inferred can never be seen directly. Elementary particles, for instance, can never be perceived directly, only inferred on the basis of effects they produce, such as tracks in a bubble chamber. To cite one example, in 1931, Paul Dirac theoretically predicted, on the basis of mathematical analyses, the existence of the elementary particle known as a positron. In the following year, Carl D. Anderson allegedly confirmed this "virtual" knowledge, or plausible hypothesis, by observing tracks produced by a particle with the qualities attributed to the predicted positron. But since only the macroscopic *effects* of positrons, and not the positrons themselves, are accessible to perception, how do we know that those effects could not possibly have been produced by something else? Of course, we could simply *define* that which produces such effects as a positron, but this reduces the objective existence of a positron to a mere convention.

Edward Wilson responds to this general problem by declaring, "Investigators think out every possible way the process might occur—the multiple competing hypotheses—and devise tests that will eliminate all but one."[55] As attractive as this notion is to proponents of scientific realism, it ignores the problem of underdetermination: the principle that for any given body of evidence, multiple, incompatible theories can be devised to account for the imperceptible causal processes that produced that evidence.[56] According to Buddhist logic, while Neptune would be classified as a hidden object prior to the time of Galileo, when he saw the appearance of Neptune, he misidentified it; but in 1846, it was correctly perceived for what it is. Thus, the earlier mathematical inference of the existence of this planet was validated by direct perception. But in the case of elementary particles and all the other so-called theoretical entities of modern physics, such perceptual validation never occurs. Thus, according to Buddhist logic, there is no valid knowledge through inference of such objects that can never be perceived. In James's terminology, all such knowledge must be deemed "virtual" at best.

All scientific observations take place with the use of specific systems of measurement and are understood within specific conceptual frameworks. On what grounds, then, can one justifiably posit the existence of objects independently of all systems of measurement and conceptual frameworks? Again, Werner Heisenberg, Max Born, and other pioneers in the field of quantum mechanics were insistent that one must not attribute existence to that which cannot be known *even in principle*. This position seems to be reflected in Buddhist thought as well. For instance, the Buddhist Sanskrit term *jñeya*, meaning "the knowable," is used interchangeably with the term *astitā*, meaning "the existent." The implication is that one should posit the existence of only that which can in principle be known by either perception or inference. This raises profound problems for asserting the existence of purely objective phenomena that allegedly produce all the appearances of the external world.[57]

The primary reason in Buddhism for using logic to infer hidden objects is to eventually extend the scope of one's perceptual knowledge. The scientific parallel is the use of retroductive logic, applied, for example, in the discovery of Neptune, which ideally leads to empirical confirmation of the inferred object. For either Buddhist or scientific reasoning to lead to inferential knowledge, one must have valid knowledge of the elements referred to in the reasoning. For example, in order to mathematically infer the presence of Neptune, one must have clear knowledge of the nature of mass, force, gravity, and the principles of Newtonian mechanics. Otherwise, no inference can be made on the basis of such mathematical reasoning.

Buddhist philosophers such as Dharmakīrti present various arguments to prove the existence of hidden entities such as former and later lives.[58] Such reasoning allegedly goes hand in hand with experiential, contemplative discoveries of the luminous, cognizant nature of consciousness as an immaterial process. Thus, when Dharmakīrti refers to consciousness or the mind in his arguments to demonstrate the continuity of individual consciousness from one life to the next, his audience must have valid, perceptual knowledge of the nature of consciousness to be able to make the inference he is suggesting. But the origins, nature, and role of consciousness in nature presently remain hidden from the investigations of scientists and philosophers. And without comprehending the nature of the mind and consciousness, one cannot make valid inferences on the basis of Dharmakīrti's philosophy.

Contrary to the conclusion of Buddhologist Roger Jackson,[59] Dharmakīrti's reasoning here requires not the unquestioning assumption of his assertions about the nature of consciousness, but valid knowledge that his hypotheses are true. However, unless one is an advanced contemplative who has experientially put those hypotheses to the test, such knowledge may remain inaccessible. On the other hand, why should anyone believe that Buddhist contemplative observations regarding the mind are valid? This requires returning to the threefold criteria for conventional existence described above. In short, these observations should be tested relative to other modes of knowledge, which is precisely how to validate empirical observations in scientific research. In both cases, investigators rely not only on their own observations and analyses but also on those of professional peers and predecessors. This brings us to the role of authority in both Buddhism and science.

INFERENTIAL KNOWLEDGE OF VERY HIDDEN OBJECTS

In the modern West, science and religion have taken radically different stances regarding truth claims based upon authority. Galileo insisted that biblical references to the natural world had to be freshly interpreted in light of the empirical and theoretical discoveries of science. Whenever scientific discoveries refuted assertions of the Bible or the tradition of medieval Christian scholasticism, the latter had to give way. The Roman Catholic Church was not so willing to relinquish its authority regarding the nature of the universe, and the rift between science and religion widened. Taking a position similar to Galileo's critique of the Church, Buddhist logicians attack other Indian philosophical traditions for relying on scriptural authority in matters that should be decided by objective inference, or the power of reason.[60] It is legitimate to resort to authority, they argue, only when the object of inquiry is not accessible to either direct perception or objective inference.

According to the two most seminal figures in the history of Buddhist logic, Dignāga (fifth century) and Dharmakīrti, in addition to evident phenomena that can be apprehended by means of perception and hidden objects that can be known by means of objective inference, there is also a class of very hidden (atyantaparokṣa) objects that can be known only by means of inference based upon authority. Once again it is important to note that hidden objects are not imperceptible *by nature*, they are hidden only relative to specific perceptual vantage points. Likewise, very hidden objects are not intrinsically inaccessible to perception or objective inference; their status is also relative to the cognitive limitations of specific individuals and communities under specific circumstances.

Let us take a specific example. As I gaze out my window while talking to my friend George on the telephone, I see his young son Tom fall off his bicycle and begin to cry, and I tell George that his son is in pain. Tom's pain is directly perceived by himself as an evident phenomenon. For me, his pain is a hidden object that I detect by means of objective inference (I perceive his crying and other behavior indicative of experiencing pain). For George, who knows me to be a truthful person with my senses intact, Tom's pain is very hidden (he can't hear Tom's crying or watch his behavior as he rises from the pavement), but he can still have inferential knowledge of it based upon my observation of Tom's behavior and my report to George. In this case, a single phenomenon—Tom's pain—is evident, hidden, and very hidden, relative to three different cognitive frames of reference.

None of these frames of reference is infallible: maybe Tom isn't really in pain, but he believes he is since he fell off his bike; maybe Tom isn't really in pain, but he wants to draw attention and sympathy to himself; and maybe Tom isn't really crying, only shouting, or I am lying to George for reasons unbeknownst to him. Nevertheless, there is a general gradation of reliability from these three vantage points: Tom is in the best position to know whether he is really in pain, and my objective inference of his pain is more reliable and informative than George's knowledge based solely on my verbal report.

In Buddhism, as in Christianity, the primary examples of very hidden realities are the truthfulness and significance of accounts in the sacred texts. In Buddhism, the authority behind such texts is enlightened beings such as the historical Buddha and a hundred generations of later Buddhist contemplative adepts. In Christianity, it is the Old Testament prophets, Jesus, his Apostles, or later authorities within the Christian tradition, all tracing their authority back to God. In both Buddhism and science, empirical knowledge is regarded as more dependable than objective inference alone, and knowledge based upon others' testimony is seen as the least reliable of these three modes of knowledge. But in both fields, the pursuit of knowledge must be based in part upon the testimony of others.[61]

In the Buddhist context, which individuals are justifiably deemed to speak with authority about matters that are generally hidden from both direct perception and objective inference? Gautama Buddha is most widely regarded by Buddhists as having the most authoritative insight into even the subtlest aspects of existence. Only a buddha, for example, is said to have the ability to directly perceive the subtle relationships between actions and their results over the course of lifetimes. Such relationships are said to be very hidden, but they are in principle observable if one achieves the spiritual awakening of a buddha. Furthermore, many scholars and contemplatives who came after the historical Buddha are also regarded as authorities (*pramāṇapuruṣa*) by specific Buddhist traditions. According to the Indo-Tibetan tradition, people with "sharp faculties" place their confidence in specific individuals on the basis of their compelling reports of their insights or their outstanding scholarship. People of "dull faculties," on the other hand, place their confidence in specific treatises or scriptures on the basis of faith in the authors of those works and their life stories.

In the scientific context as well, specific individuals throughout history have been deemed authorities. Newton, Maxwell, and Einstein are examples who immediately spring to mind, but there are many others, including the recipients of numerous Nobel prizes in the various sciences. In addition, award-winning scientists holding endowed chairs at prestigious institutions of research and higher education are widely believed to speak with greater authority than people lacking such credentials. While physicists may hold Einstein in awe for the elegance and profundity of his theories in the fields of special and general relativity, as well as quantum mechanics, nonscientists are more likely to regard his theories as authoritative because he—the most celebrated genius of the twentieth century—devised them. Here is the parallel with the Buddhist distinction between individuals of sharp and dull faculties. But there are also important differences between the Buddhist and scientific attitudes toward authority. Traditional Buddhists do not question the fundamental authenticity of the Buddha's enlightenment and the insights that came with it, though they may certainly question *their understanding* of those insights. Scientists, on the other hand, regard no individual scientist or scientific theory to be ultimately authoritative. Newton's assumptions about absolute space and time have been proven false, as have Einstein's assumptions about locality in the realm of quantum mechanics. Practicing Buddhists seek to replicate in their own experience the spiritual awakening of the Buddha, while scientists seek to make unprecedented advances in the pursuit of objective knowledge. This is a crucial difference between the two disciplines.

In the Indo-Tibetan Buddhist tradition, clear criteria are presented for determining which treatises can be deemed to be authoritative, which is to say that they can be used as bases for making sound inferences based upon the testimony of others. Such a treatise must be unrefuted by valid perception, unrefuted by objective inference, and free from contradiction with other propositions whose truth is textually inferred.[62] The third criterion implies a kind of circularity in reasoning reminiscent of the previously discussed threefold criteria for establishing conventional existence. One way out of this circularity, in both Buddhism and science, is to take into account pragmatic as well as epistemic factors in determining who or what is real or authoritative. As Dharmakīrti writes, treatises are worth investigating when they present coherent, practicable methods for gaining results, specifically in terms of the experiential realization of spiritual goals.[63] Moreover, when a certain individual's words have been found to be correct regarding some aspects of reality that were previously hidden, this gives grounds for confidence that the same person may speak authoritatively about other matters beyond one's own present knowledge. But of course there is no guarantee for either Buddhist contemplatives or scientists.

A Buddhist contemplative who has gained deep insights into the nature of the mind may be radically mistaken in his understanding of brain functions; and a neuroscientist who is conducting cutting-edge research on the brain may be radically mistaken about the nature of consciousness. Nevertheless, neither aspiring contemplatives nor scientists are likely to make much progress if they do not rely upon the authoritative empirical reports and theoretical analyses of their most distinguished predecessors. In the Indo-Tibetan Buddhist tradition, such treatises are subject to peer review by other contemplatives and scholars, and in the scientific tradition, research papers and books are subject to peer review in professional journals and academic presses.

In both science and Buddhism, researchers have the option of drawing inferences based upon the authoritative testimonies of their predecessors and peers. If Buddhist contemplatives disregarded all such reports, their progress toward spiritual awakening would be radically impaired; and if scientists refused to rely upon the reports of the engineers who create their technology or the findings of other scientists, scientific progress would slow to a snail's pace. Those dedicated to discovering truth—by means of either contemplative or scientific inquiry—accept as *working hypotheses* the authoritative assertions of others regarding objects that are presently very hidden from themselves.

People not interested in testing Buddhist techniques for developing meditative concentration and contemplative insights do not need to accept as working hypotheses Buddhist assertions regarding the plasticity of attention and the potentials of introspective inquiry. Those who are not concerned with achieving favorable rebirth or spiritual awakening as conceived in Buddhism do not need to accept Buddhist theories regarding the nature of consciousness as their working hypotheses. Similarly, nonscientists who are not interested in how the universe operates are under no obligation to accept any scientific assertions as their working hypotheses. Anyone can ignore or dismiss all truth claims made by contemplatives and scientists about very hidden objects. But in accepting only what they personally know to be true and accepting nothing as a working hypothesis, they tie themselves into a very small knot in the vast fabric of human knowledge.

CONCLUSION

Regarding the three modes of knowledge—perception, objective inference, and inference based on authority—empiricists, including many scientists and Buddhist contemplatives, most highly value perception; rationalists, including many philosophers, both Western and Buddhist, most highly value logical inference; and dogmatists, including many scientific materialists and religious believers, most highly value inference based on authority. In the final category, scientific materialists adhere to the principles of their dogma, regardless of conflicting evidence. Any such evidence is not even counted *because it does not conform to their metaphysical principles.* Likewise, dogmatic Buddhists cling tenaciously to the validity of their scriptures or traditions, attributing to them an infallibility that is immune to both empirical evidence and logical reasoning.

Buddhism is commonly categorized as a religion—a view that hides its empirical and rational elements—on the grounds that the vast majority of Buddhists relate to it as such. Its principles are accepted on authority, without concern for empirically or rationally corroborating them for oneself. But this is precisely how the vast majority of the lay public who believe in science accepts its discoveries and theories. Scientific assertions are accepted by most people on the basis of authority. The major difference between such followers of Buddhism and followers of science is their choice of authorities.

If my previous analysis of objective knowledge is correct, scientists cannot validate their claim to have discovered truths about the universe independent of their systems of measurement and conceptual frameworks. But this assertion does not necessarily imply a retreat into cultural relativism. Rather, science has unveiled countless intersubjective truths about the natural world that are invariant across multiple cognitive frames of reference. That is, it has revealed facts that are true not only for all human beings but also for all other known species of sentient beings. To be sure, science has repudiated many of its most cherished theories and conclusions over the past four centuries, and scientists still disagree with one another on a wide variety of fronts. But they also agree on many points, and their knowledge has provided enormous pragmatic benefits, especially in the advances of medicine and technology.

Diversity of experiential insights and theoretical interpretations is also very common among the many traditions of Buddhism, not to mention other, non-Buddhist contemplative traditions. While it seems implausible to validate any one while discrediting all the others, I would argue that it is just as unreasonable to invalidate all of them, simply because they differ among themselves. Perhaps it can be helpful to take an analogy from the history of physics. *Ontologically*, the laws of classical physics—with their underlying assumptions of absolute space and time and the independent, local existence of individual elementary particles—are incorrect at all speeds and for all sizes of phenomena. But *pragmatically*, calculations based on classical physics—without taking into consideration either relativity theory or quantum theory—are the most useful for understanding and controlling a wide range of macrophenomena moving at nonrelativistic velocities. Likewise, for some purposes it may be perfectly adequate to view light (or any other physical phenomenon) simply as a particle or as a wave. But the more deeply one probes the actual nature of physical reality at its most fundamental level, the less useful are the crude and partial assumptions and models of classical physics.

Likewise, different, mutually incompatible Buddhist views may be pragmatically useful for specific people who are practicing at relatively elementary levels of contemplative insight. To draw a parallel with physics, the laws of classical mechanics are pragmatically useful for understanding the behavior of slow-moving, macroscopic bodies, but the theories of relativity and quantum mechanics show the provisional nature of those laws. Twentieth-century physics casts fresh light on the nature of bodies moving at or near the speed of light and of elementary particles and waves. These insights challenge us to reframe our overall understanding of the physical world at large, a point often lost on scientists working in the fields of biology and psychology. An assumption that is pragmatically useful in one arena may be profoundly misleading in terms of understanding nature as a whole.

Addressing this issue from another angle, differences in views among scientists, among Buddhists, or between scientists and Buddhists may be adopted from roughly the same perspective, but may turn out to be complementary rather than simply conflicting. On the other hand, the *apparent* differences in opposing views may be due to their being adopted from radically different perspectives. There may also be *real* differences in views that purport to speak from roughly the same perspective (e.g., a God's-eye view or a purely objective view from nowhere, which is oblivious to any subjective perspective), but draw different conclusions. Such problems call for detailed analysis to understand the nature of differences in scientific and Buddhist assertions. At the same time, it is important not to overlook insights that may be common to science and Buddhism, as well as other contemplative traditions. For these truths, which are invariant over radically different cognitive frames of reference, may be very deep and significant for humanity as a whole.

One fundamental difference between the scientific pursuit of objective truth and the Buddhist pursuit of spiritual awakening is that the former has relied principally on third-person modes of investigating external, physical phenomena, while the latter has relied primarily on first-person modes of investigating internal, mental phenomena. If all mental phenomena are in fact merely epiphenomena, or emergent processes, of physical events that occurred very late in the evolution of the universe, then scientists, not Buddhists, would speak with the greatest authority about the nature of the mind. But modern science has yet to devise any means of objectively studying the origins, nature, or role of consciousness in nature, either at present or over the billions of years since the Big Bang. Since scientists have no way of objectively detecting the presence of consciousness in any sentient being now—even those we know firsthand to be conscious—they certainly cannot claim to know whether consciousness of any kind existed in the distant past. If, as Buddhists claim, consciousness is at least as fundamental to the universe as mass-energy and space-time, then it is plausible that the deep exploration of consciousness might reveal truths about the objective world as well as the subjective, even truths concerning the origins of the universe. This is a question to be explored empirically, with as few metaphysical biases as possible. The way forward in any fruitful collaboration between Buddhism and science is by letting go of subjective, ideological biases of all kinds, and uniting forces in the pursuit of empirical discoveries and open-minded, rational inquiry.

5

BUDDHIST NONTHEISM,
POLYTHEISM, AND MONOTHEISM

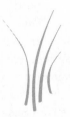

FOR A VARIETY of reasons Buddhism is usually referred to as a nontheistic religion, and this sets it radically apart from Christianity and all other theistic religions. Scholars may classify Buddhism in this way simply to point out one of its differences. Theists may do so to show the inferiority of Buddhism compared to their own creed; conversely, Buddhists may emphasize its nontheistic status as a means of demonstrating its superiority. There are certainly plenty of experts in the field of Buddhist studies who express this view. For instance, shortly after his conversion from Buddhism to Christianity, Buddhologist Paul Williams declared, "*All* Buddhism is actually atheism, whatever is said sometimes nowadays about its being agnostic."[1]

However, contrary to this widespread classification, upon more careful examination, various Buddhist traditions appear to be nontheistic, polytheistic, and even monotheistic. Williams is correct, though, in refuting those who make the indefensible claim that Buddhism is agnostic.[2]

THE QUASI-ATHEISTIC STATUS OF THERAVĀDA BUDDHISM

Among the earliest Buddhist sources cited to establish Buddhism as nontheistic is the Buddha's own assertion that the world was not brought into existence by a divine creator or by chance.[3] In the Buddhist view, it is not the god Brahmā but the actions, or karma, of sentient beings, individually and collectively, that give rise to the myriad worlds of experience (*loka*). Karma, it is said, ripens as subjective experiences of pleasure and pain and as felicitous and adverse circumstances. However, karma is not thought to be responsible for everything that occurs in nature, such as apples falling from trees or iron filings moving toward a magnet.[4]

While there are ample writings in the Pāli Buddhist canon (Pāli being the language in which the Buddha's teachings were first recorded) illustrating that Theravāda Buddhism refutes the existence of an independent creator who rules the world, such assertions in no way imply that Buddhism does away with gods altogether. Indeed, given the countless references to a wide range of gods of the desire, form, and formless realms, Buddhism can rightly be classified as polytheistic. Simply put, the desire realm consists of the world of the physical senses, to which sentient beings respond with desire for agreeable objects and aversion to the disagreeable. The form realm is a more subtle dimension of pure forms and archetypes, and the formless realm is a purely abstract domain of reality that transcends all forms. In the earliest accounts of the Buddha's enlightenment, the gods Indra and Brahmā are said to have requested the Buddha to teach, to turn the wheel of Dharma. And throughout the *sūtras*, *tantras*, and authoritative commentaries by Buddhist scholars over the ages, there are detailed descriptions of a multitude of gods inhabiting the universe and influencing natural events, such as the weather and the lives of individuals. To this day, there are widespread practices of worshipping and propitiating gods throughout virtually all Buddhist traditions in Southeast, East, and Central Asian schools of Buddhism.

Such polytheism is absent primarily among modern Western converts. The affirmation of such gods and their inclusion in spiritual practice has always been of secondary importance in Buddhism, so most Western Buddhists have skipped or marginalized this aspect. But it is a categorical error to state that all Buddhism is atheistic, when it so undeniably affirms the existence of a whole pantheon of gods.

When Paul Williams declares Buddhism to be totally atheistic, he is stressing a dramatic contrast with the monotheism of Christianity. Nowhere is this distinction more obvious than between Christianity and Theravāda Buddhism. According to this school, the ground state of consciousness from which all active mental processes arise (*javana*) is known as the *bhavaṅga*, the ground of becoming, which bears a striking resemblance to the substrate consciousness discussed earlier.[5] As the basis of all mental activities, the *bhavaṅga* is the source of karma and hence of the phenomenal world experienced by each sentient being. Such a view is presented as an alternative to the monotheistic belief in a single, independent creator who made and rules the phenomenal world. The *bhavaṅga* is an individual continuum of consciousness to which the Buddha referred when he declared, "Monks, this mind is brightly shining, but it is defiled by adventitious defilements. Monks, this mind is brightly shining, and it is free from adventitious defilements."[6] It is said that this dimension of consciousness arouses one to develop one's mind through meditation,[7] and with the attainment of liberation, the *bhavaṅga* retains its integrity and is no longer prone to obscuration by defilements. While the normal functioning of consciousness is like light, which may get cut off, the *bhavaṅga* has a radiance that exists whether or not it is obscured.

The theory of the *bhavaṅga* is presented not as a product of mystical speculation but as a phenomenological account of a state of consciousness realized through the cultivation of meditative stabilization (*jhāna*), beginning with the achievement of *śamatha*. The modern Theravāda scholar Paravahera Vajirañāṇa writes:[8]

> Just as a baby, when placed upon its feet, falls down repeatedly, even so the mind in access-samādhi remains for a moment upon the object of Paṭibhāga [counterpart sign] and then lapses into Bhavaṅga, the state of its primal being or subconscious flow. But once the mind has risen from Bhavaṅga to the height of Appaṇā-samādhi, which is very strong because it is associated with the Jhāna factors, it may remain upon the object for a whole day and a night, where it proceeds by way of a succession of wholesome thoughts.

In the Pāli canon a parallel is drawn between dying and going to sleep.[9] Dreamless sleep is presented as a state of uninterrupted *bhavaṅga*,[10] which is also the very last state of consciousness prior to death.[11] Again the parallels with the substrate consciousness as described in the Great Perfection school are remarkable, especially in light of the fact that these two traditions of Buddhism have had very little contact over the centuries.

While it is commonly said of the Mahāyāna tradition that it deified the Buddha as an omnipresent, divine consciousness, the Pāli canon is notably silent on the status of the Buddha after his *parinirvāṇa*.[12] In one often-quoted dialogue, when asked whether a buddha exists, does not exist, both exists and doesn't exist, or neither exists nor doesn't exist after death, the Buddha responded with "noble silence," choosing instead to discuss the Four Noble Truths, which he felt were more pertinent to the spiritual needs of the questioner.[13] A common interpretation of his silence is that all four of the logical options presented to him are expressions of conceptual elaborations concerning existence and nonexistence; and none applies to the Buddha after his passing. All such conceptual elaborations are inadequate and misleading in this regard.

Theravāda Buddhist literature does, however, comment that at death the Buddha was like a flame of a great mass of fire that goes out, "gone beyond designation."[14] Many people have interpreted this to mean that the Buddha ceased to exist, contrary to the implication of his noble silence on this matter. However, the authors of this Buddhist assertion, like those of the Hindu Upaniṣads, took for granted a quiescent, nonburning form of fire, "an indestructible element latent in every bright or warm thing, but especially in fuel. It alternates between manifestation and 'going home' to its occult source."[15]

In seeking to distance itself from non-Buddhist Indian philosophical systems, the Theravāda tradition has gone out of its way to emphasize the non-existence of God and immortal souls. While all Buddhist schools refute the existence of an immutable, unitary, independent self, this does not mean that there is no continuity of an individual stream of consciousness after death. Indeed, this seems indispensable if Buddhists are to accept the theory of karma and reincarnation taught in the Pāli canon, which also refers to the existence of an intermediate phase of conscious experience following death and prior to one's next incarnation (*antarā-bhava*).[16] But the Theravāda tradition has come to marginalize the evidence in its own scriptures that assert such an intermediate period, possibly because this might be seen as incompatible with its refutation of a independent self (*ātman*). Likewise, presenting strong opposition to the theistic theories of other Indian systems of thought, Theravāda Buddhism has come to regard the Buddha after his death as being nonexistent *for all practical purposes*, despite the fact that its own scriptures declare that his status transcends all conceptual designations.

THE QUASI-MONOTHEISTIC STATUS
OF MAHĀYĀNA BUDDHISM

Like Theravāda Buddhism, the Mahāyāna tradition, which emerged around the beginning of the Common Era, also refutes the existence of a god who created and rules the world. For instance, Śāntideva presented a detailed argument in refutation of Īśvara as the divine creator of the world.[17] Like earlier generations of Buddhist scholars, he took great pains to point out important distinctions among the views of his own Buddhist school, other Buddhist schools, and non-Buddhist Indian traditions. The refutation of a creator was seen as a key point in differentiating Buddhist from non-Buddhist views.

All schools of Mahāyāna Buddhism also refute the existence of an immutable, unitary, independent self. However, in its assertions of the intrinsic purity of the luminous consciousness of each sentient being (*tathāgatagarbha*) and of the omnipresent, divine consciousness of the Buddha (*dharmakāya*), the Mahāyāna diverges in some important respects from the Theravāda theory of the ground state of each individual's consciousness prior to enlightenment and its ultimate status after achieving enlightenment. While embracing the relative polytheism of the Buddhism presented in the Pāli canon, it abandons the pragmatic atheism of Theravāda Buddhism, accepting in its place a view that may be deemed quasi-monotheistic.

In a manner reminiscent of the Pāli canon's version of the *bhavaṅga*, the *Aṣṭasāhasrikā Perfection of Wisdom Sūtra* refers to the mind of a *bodhisattva*, known as the spirit of awakening (*bodhicitta*), when it asserts "that mind is no mind, since it is by nature brightly shining."[18] The *Laṅkāvatāra Sūtra* similarly asserts that the buddha-nature (*tathāgatagarbha*) is "brightly shining and pure, and originally pure, but it appears impure as it is defiled by adventitious stains and is enveloped by the *skandhas*, *dhātus*, and soiled with the dirt of attachment, hatred, delusion, and compulsive ideation."[19] In reference to this primordial dimension of consciousness, the *sūtra* declares that it "holds within it the cause for both good and evil, and by it all forms of existence are produced. Like an actor it takes on a variety of forms."[20]

Another Mahāyāna *sūtra*, the *Śrīmālā-devī Siṃhanāda Sūtra*, states that the buddha-nature is that which arouses one to aspire for *nirvāṇa*; and, like the *Laṅkāvatāra Sūtra*, states that this consciousness is not the self. On the other hand, the *Mahāparinirvāṇa-sūtra* declares that the buddha-nature is nothing other than the self:[21] "I do not say that all sentient beings lack a Self. I always say that sentient beings have the Buddha-nature (*svabhāva*). Is not that very Buddha-nature a Self? So I do not teach a nihilistic doctrine."[22] The *Ratnagotra-vibhāga*, an influential Mahāyāna Buddhist treatise attributed to the Bodhisattva Maitreya, declares that the buddha-nature is replete with the qualities of Buddhahood.[23] The Chinese version of the *Ratnagotra-vibhāga* explains the *Mahāparinirvāṇa-sūtra*'s references to self by stating that the Buddha has a True Self (*shih-wo*), which is beyond being and nonbeing. In other words, it transcends all conceptual elaborations (*prapañca*). While the intrinsically pure and luminous buddha-nature is naturally present since beginningless time, the *Ratnagotra-vibhāga* states that it is to be "perfected through proper cultivation."[24] According to this tradition, it is not only the ground of each individual's mental activities, karma, and experience but also the basis of all existence.[25] This view seems to be in complete conformity with the Great Perfection theory of primordial consciousness, which is explicitly equated with the buddha-nature.

Closely related to the Mahāyāna theory of the buddha-nature is its description of the mind of the Buddha (*dharmakāya*), which goes far beyond any description found in the Pāli canon. According to one Mahāyāna *sūtra*, the two are essentially equated with each other: "This Dharmakāya of the Tathāgatas when not free from the store of defilement is referred to as the Tathāgatagarbha."[26] The *dharmakāya* is described as beginningless, unborn, undying, permanent, and possessed of innumerable good qualities. Intrinsically pure, radiant consciousness, it is the ground and ultimate nature of the entire universe. According to the *Ratnagotra-vibhāga*, the *dharmakāya* nondually pervades the minds of all unenlightened and enlightened beings alike, and its nature is pure, radiant, all-pervasive consciousness.[27] While there are innumerable buddhas, manifesting in myriad forms throughout the universe, there is but one *dharmakāya*, so the minds of all the buddhas are undifferentiated, transcending the conceptual divisions of "one" and "many."

The experiential realization of the ultimate nonduality of one's own *tathāgatagarbha* and the *dharmakāya* is of paramount importance in Mahāyāna Buddhism. While the *dharmakāya* is said to transcend all conceptual elaborations, including the categories of existence and nonexistence, for all practical purposes, the Mahāyāna tradition regards the buddha-mind as existent throughout all time. In this regard, one may speak of the "living Buddha" in much the same way that Christians speak of the "living Christ."[28] For Mahāyāna Buddhists worship the Buddha as a divine presence here and now, much as Christians worship Christ. In this context, the Buddha is clearly viewed as a supreme deity to whom they make supplicatory prayers and from whom they believe they receive blessings and guidance. While Mahāyāna Buddhism refutes certain notions of the self and a divine creator, it clearly does not do away with the self or a supreme deity altogether, so it may best be described as quasi-monotheistic.

THE MONOTHEISTIC STATUS OF VAJRAYĀNA BUDDHISM

As in the Theravāda and Mahāyāna traditions, nontheistic trends appear in Vajrayāna Buddhist sources, which emerged during the early centuries of the Common Era. For example, the *Kālacakratantra* (which did not appear in India until the eleventh century) and its principal commentary, the *Vimalaprabhā*, lay out rational arguments to refute Īśvara as the creator.[29] The *Vimalaprabhā* states, "Everything animate and inanimate comes into existence due to the agglomeration of substances. The nature of karma is not due to the Creator's will. This is a universal rule."[30] This tantric treatise further argues that there is no independent creator who governs the world or punishes sin and rewards virtue. Instead, it explains the vicissitudes of life in terms of dependent origination (*pratītya-samutpāda*) in accordance with the Madhyamaka view.

Nevertheless, the theories of the *tathāgatagarbha* and the *dharmakāya* play a central role in Vajrayāna Buddhism. In the Mahāyāna tradition, there are treatises that present the *tathāgatagarbha* simply as a capacity for enlightenment, which is to be developed through strenuous practice. Other Mahāyāna sources describe it as a present reality, replete with all the qualities of Buddhahood, but temporarily veiled by mental obscurations. But a central feature of Vajrayāna practice, known as the cultivation of "pure vision," is to simulate what could be called a "God's-eye view of reality," seeking to view all phenomena from the perspective of a buddha. Thus, the *tathāgatagarbha* is regarded not simply as a potential but as a manifest reality, here and now. Yet it is paradoxically asserted to transcend all conceptual elaborations.

The Theravāda tradition asserts that the *bhavaṅga* is dormant when the active mind is aroused, yet it is the *bhavaṅga* that motivates one to seek *nirvāṇa*, and it is the basis of all the phenomena that appear to the senses. Likewise, some Mahāyāna and Vajrayāna interpretations of the *tathāgatagarbha* assert it is dormant when the dualistic mind is active, yet the *tathāgatagarbha* still arouses one to seek enlightenment and acts as the basis of existence. But according to the Great Perfection school of Vajrayāna Buddhism, the *tathāgatagarbha* is viewed as saturating all mental states and processes, even those that are afflictive and delusional. As such, it is nondual from the *dharmakāya*, which pervades the whole of *saṃsāra* and *nirvāṇa*.

In Vajrayāna Buddhism in general, and the Great Perfection school in particular, the *dharmakāya* is variously personified as Samantabhadra, Vajradhara, and the Ādibuddha, or Primordial Buddha, the source of all phenomena, yet it is not different from the buddha-nature of each sentient being. In this regard, the *Kālacakratantra* states, "Apart from sentient beings there is no great Buddha."[31] This postulation of the Ādibuddha unifies the early Buddhist theory that sentient beings create the worlds in which they dwell, and the Vajrayāna theory that the universe has its source in the Ādibuddha.

As the early Buddhist theory of the *bhavaṅga* was a precursor to the Mahāyāna theory of the *tathāgatagarbha*, the precise manner in which the *tathāgatagarbha* gives rise to the phenomenal world was further developed in the Vajrayāna tradition. My primary source for the following account of Vajrayāna cosmogony is *The Vajra Essence*, a nineteenth-century "mind-treasure" (*dgongs gter*) of Düdjom Lingpa.[32] Although this treatise is of relatively recent origin, its theory of cosmogony is an accurate representation of the Great Perfection view, which, in turn, is largely compatible with Vajrayāna theory as a whole. According to Düdjom Lingpa, the source of the teachings in *The Vajra Essence* is the primordial Buddha Samantabhadra, who, like the *tathāgatagarbha*, is of the nature of beginningless, naturally pure, radiant awareness, replete with all the qualities of Buddhahood.

While the most common metaphor for the *bhavaṅga* and the *tathāgatagarbha* is that of radiant light, *The Vajra Essence* adds the central metaphor of space. According to this cosmogony, the essential nature of the whole of reality is the absolute space of phenomena, but this space is not to be confused with a mere absence of matter. Rather, it is imbued with all the infinite knowledge, compassion, power, and enlightened activities of the Buddha. Moreover, this luminous space is that which causes the phenomenal world to appear, and it is none other than the nature of one's own mind, which is clear light.[33] Samantabhadra distinguishes five facets of primordial consciousness implicit within the natural buddha of awareness:[34]

Its essential nature is primordial, great emptiness, the absolute space of the whole of *saṃsāra* and *nirvāṇa*, the primordial consciousness of the absolute space of phenomena. Mirror-like primordial consciousness is of a limpid, clear nature free of contamination, which allows for the unceasing appearances of all manner of objects. The primordial consciousness of equality is so called, for it equally pervades the nonobjective emptiness of the whole of *saṃsāra* and *nirvāṇa*. The primordial consciousness of discernment is so called, for it is an unceasing avenue of illumination of the qualities of primordial consciousness. The primordial consciousness of accomplishment is so called, for all pure, free, simultaneously perfected deeds and activities are accomplished naturally, of their own accord. When the natural glow of awareness that is present as the ground—the *dharmakāya* in which the five facets of primordial consciousness are simultaneously perfected—dissolves into its inner luminosity, it is classified as *unobscured primordial* consciousness.

SETS OF FIVE

PRIMORDIAL CONSCIOUSNESS	GREAT ELEMENT	DERIVATIVE ELEMENT	AGGREGATE	POISON
absolute space of phenomena	blue	space	form	delusion
mirrorlike	white	water	consciousness	hatred
equality	yellow	earth	feeling	pride
discernment	red	fire	recognition	attachment
accomplishment	green	air	compositional factors	envy

If the essential nature of each sentient being and the universe as a whole is infinite, luminous space, endowed with all the qualities of perfect enlightenment, why is this not realized? Samantabhadra explains that the reality of all phenomena arising as displays of the all-pervasive ground awareness is obscured by ignorance. Consequently, the *tathāgatagarbha*, which utterly transcends all words and concepts—including the very notions of existence and nonexistence, one and many, and subject and object—is experientially reduced to a blank, unthinking void, which is known as the substrate (*ālaya*). The experience of this void is comparable to becoming comatose or falling into dreamless sleep, totally lacking in content. From that state arises limpid, clear consciousness as the basis from which all phenomena appear, and that is the substrate consciousness (*ālayavijñāna*). No objects are established apart from its own luminosity, and while it produces all types of appearances, it does not enter into any object. Just as reflections of the planets and stars appear in limpid, clear water and the entire animate and inanimate world appears in limpid, clear space, so do all appearances appear in the empty, clear, universal ground consciousness.

From that state arises the consciousness of the mere appearance of the self. The self, or "I," is apprehended as being "here," so the objective world seems to be "over there," thus establishing the appearance of space. To relate this evolution of the universe to the obscuration of the previously mentioned five facets of primordial consciousness, it is said that ignorance initially obscures the inner glow of one's innate, primordial consciousness of the absolute space of reality, which causes an external transference of its radiance. As this evolutionary process continues, the five types of primordial consciousness transform into the five great elements and the five derivative elements in the following way:

1. In the all-pervasive space of the *dharmakāya*, the inner glow of the primordial consciousness of accomplishment is obscured, and due to the activation of karmic energies, the quintessence of the air element arises internally and transforms into radiant green light. Due to the power of delusion, this green light is reified and consequently arises externally as the derivative, or residual, air element.

2. With the obscuration by ignorance of the primordial consciousness of the absolute space of phenomena, its radiance appears as the great element of deep blue light. As a consequence of reifying this blue light, the derivative element of space appears.

3. With the obscuration of mirrorlike primordial consciousness, its radiance appears as the great element of white light, which, when reified, appears as the derivative element of water.

4. With the obscuration of the primordial consciousness of equality, its radiance appears as the great element of yellow light, which, when reified, appears as the derivative element of earth.

5. Finally, with the obscuration of the primordial consciousness of discernment, its radiance appears as the great element of red light, which, when reified, appears as the derivative element of fire. In this way, all the elements of the physical world are regarded as symbolic expressions of the *tathāgatgarbha*, and all the five elements are said to be present in each one, just as all five facets of primordial consciousness are present in each one.

The five facets of primordial consciousness manifest as the five elements that make up the objective universe, and their essential natures also manifest as the five psycho-physical aggregates that constitute a human being in *saṃsāra*. Specifically, once the appearance of duality arises within the domain of the primordial consciousness of the absolute space of reality, that wisdom appears as the aggregate of form; when such dualistic appearances and reification occur in the domain of mirrorlike primordial consciousness, it manifests as the aggregate of consciousness; when the primordial consciousness of equality is so obscured, it manifests as the aggregate of feeling; when the primordial consciousness of discernment is veiled by reification, it appears as the aggregate of recognition; and when the primordial consciousness of accomplishment is so obscured, it arises as the aggregate of compositional factors.

As a development of the thesis stated in the *Laṅkāvatāra Sūtra,* that the *tathāgatagarbha* is the source of both good and evil, *The Vajra Essence* asserts that it is the ground not only of all the qualities of enlightenment but also of the primary mental afflictions of delusion, hatred, pride, attachment, and envy. Specifically, delusion arises due to the obscuration of the primordial consciousness of the absolute nature of reality; hatred arises from the obscuration of mirrorlike primordial consciousness; pride emerges from the obscuration of the primordial consciousness of equality; attachment emerges from the obscuration of the primordial consciousness of discernment; and envy arises from the obscuration of the primordial consciousness of accomplishment. An assertion crucial to the theory and practice of Vajrayāna as a whole is that all mental afflictions are in reality of the very same nature as the kinds of primordial consciousness from which they arise.

In summary, the five great elements, the five derivative elements, the five aggregates, and the five mental afflictions all originate from the obscuration of the five facets of primordial consciousness. In terms of the general Buddhist theory of the three realms of existence—the sensory realm, the form realm, and the formless realm—it is said that birth as a god of the sensory realm is due to achieving attentional stability in the realm of the dualistic mind (*citta*); birth in the form realm is due to reifying the substrate consciousness; and birth in the formless realm is due to reifying the substrate. In this way, Samantabhadra, the primordial Buddha whose nature is identical with the *tathāgatagarbha* within each sentient being, is the ultimate ground of *saṃsāra* and *nirvāṇa,* and the entire universe consists of nothing other than displays of this infinite, radiant, empty awareness. Thus, Vajrayāna Buddhism presents the universe as a kind of theophany, including its own version of monotheism, that may be seen as evolving from but not identical to the views of the Theravāda and Mahāyāna traditions.

The Indian contemplative Padmasambhava, who had a seminal role in introducing Vajrayāna Buddhism, and especially the Great Perfection, into Tibet in the eighth century, gave the following account of the contemplative experience of one's buddha-nature:[35]

Once you have calmed the compulsive thoughts in your mind right where they are, and the mind is unmodified, isn't there a motionless stability? Oh, this is called "quiescence," but it is not the nature of the mind. Now, steadily observe the very nature of your own mind that is being still. Is there a resplendent emptiness that is nothing, that is ungrounded in the nature of any substance, shape, or color? That is called the "empty essence." Isn't there a luster of that emptiness that is unceasing, clear, immaculate, soothing, and luminous, as it were? That is called its "luminous nature." Its essential nature is the indivisibility of sheer emptiness, not established as anything, and in its unceasing, vivid luster such awareness is resplendent and brilliant, so to speak.

Vajrayāna and Christian Traditions of Monotheism

Just as multiple, diverse theories have arisen within Buddhism, so they have in Christianity. One Christian tradition that promotes a cosmogony remarkably similar to that of Vajrayāna Buddhism is the Neoplatonic school of mysticism that was practiced in medieval Europe. According to John Scotus Eriugena, prior to God's creative self-disclosure in the generation of the natural world, he subsisted as a primordial unity and fullness that, from the limited perspective of created intellects and language, can best be described as *nihil*, or nothingness.[36] John characterized this nothingness not as an absence but as a transcendent reality beyond negation and affirmation. It is

the ineffable, incomprehensible, and inaccessible brilliance of the divine goodness, which is unknown to all intellects, whether human or angelic, because it is superessential and supernatural. I should think that this designation [*nihil*] is applied because, when it is thought through itself, it neither is nor was nor will be. For in no existing thing is it understood, since it is beyond all things.... When it is understood as incomprehensible on account of its excellence, it is not improperly called "nothing."[37]

As the divine nothingness, which is ontologically prior to the very categories of existence and nonexistence, manifests in the phenomenal world, God comes to recognize himself as the essence of all things. In this way, the whole of creation can be called a theophany, or divine appearance, and nothing can exist apart from that divine nature, for it is the essence of all that is. Following the biblical assertion that man is created in the image of God, John declares that the mind of man, like the divine nature, retains its simple unity as something that cannot be known objectively in relation to its manifold expressions. Just as God comes to know himself fully only through his self-expression as the phenomenal world, the human mind is fully comprehended only through its outward manifestations, even though it remains invisible inwardly. Each human recapitulates within himself the entire dialectic of nothingness and self-creation. Hence John argues that man's inability to objectively know the nature of his own mind marks him as being an image of

God, for just as the mind of God does not objectively see itself, so is human consciousness never perceived as an object of the intellect. This assertion is remarkably similar to the following statement in the *Ratnacūḍasūtra*:

> The mind, Kāśyapa, is formless, unseen, intangible, unknowable, unstable, un-grounded. The mind, Kāśyapa, was never seen by any of the Buddhas. They do not see it, they will not see it … the mind, Kāśyapa, being sought all around is not found: what is not found is not established; what is not established is not past, present, or future.[38]

The Neoplatonic mysticism advocated by John Scotus Eriugena domi-nated Christian thought through much of the medieval era and was pro-moted as late as the fifteenth century by Nicholas of Cusa. In arguing for the immanence of God in the human soul, Nicholas writes, "In God's light is all our knowledge, so that it is not we ourselves who know, but rather it is God who knows in us."[39] Declaring that in God all things are God, he writes, "*Theos*, who is the beginning from which everything flows forth, the middle in which we move, and the end to which everything flows back again, is everything."[40]

Much as the Mahāyāna and Vajrayāna schools of Buddhism emphasize the importance of realizing one's own buddha-nature through contemplative inquiry, Nicholas presents a comparable path of Christian contemplation:[41]

> Finally, there is still a path of seeking God within yourself: the path of the removal of limits.… When … you conceive that God is better than can be conceived, you reject everything that is limited and contracted.… If you seek further, you find nothing in yourself like God, but rather you affirm that God is above all these as the cause, beginning, and light of life of your intellective soul.… You will rejoice to have found God beyond all your interiority as the source of the good, from which everything that you have flows out to you. You turn yourself to God by entering each day more deeply within yourself and forsaking everything that lies outside in order that you be found on that path on which God is met so that after this you can apprehend God in truth.

CONCLUSION

The Vajrayāna tradition does not represent the whole of Buddhism any more than Neoplatonic Christian mysticism represents the whole of Christianity. But the same may be said of any school or tradition of either belief system. Neither is a monolithic tradition with a single, universally accepted doctrine. Differences between the two are easily found. The monotheism of mainstream Christianity that is commonly taught in churches today is a far cry from the atheism of Theravāda Buddhism that is commonly taught in Buddhist monasteries throughout Southeast Asia. But these real differences should not obscure real similarities in other traditions of Buddhism and Christianity.

The common ground in the cosmogonies outlined above may also be discovered in the Vedānta tradition and in the mystical Islamic and Jewish theories of creation influenced by the writings of Plotinus (205–270). This apparent commonality can be attributed to mere coincidence, or to the historical propagation of a single, speculative, metaphysical theory throughout South Asia and the Near East. For example, the Upaniṣads may well have influenced the writings of early Mahāyāna thinkers in India, and they could also have made their way to the Near East, where they might have inspired the writings of Plotinus. On the other hand, Plotinus declared that his theories were based on his own experiential insights, and similar claims have been made by many Buddhist, Christian, and Vedāntin contemplatives. If these cosmogonies are indeed based upon valid introspective knowledge, then there may be some plausibility to their assertions that introspective inquiry can lead to knowledge of the ultimate ground of being.

While most theologians, philosophers, and contemplatives of the world's religions throughout history have tended to emphasize the differences between their own and others' traditions, this has not invariably been the case. For instance, Padmasambhava wrote:[42]

> Astonishing! The ongoing cognizance and luminosity called the *mind* exists, but does not exist even as a single thing.... It is a label, for it is named in unimaginable ways. Some people call it the *mind-itself*. Some non-Buddhists call it the *Self*. Śrāvakas call it personal identitylessness. Cittamātrins call it the *mind*. Some people call it the *middle way*. Some call it the *perfection of wisdom*. Some give it the name *tathāgatagarbha*. Some give it the name Mahāmudrā. Some give it the name *ordinary consciousness*. Some call it the sole *bindu*. Some give it the name *dharmadhātu*. Some give it the name the *substrate*.

This integrative view, asserting a common ground to some of the deepest contemplative insights of diverse traditions despite the differences in their institutional doctrines, has come to be known in modern times as the perennial philosophy.[43] Under the domination of so much postmodern thinking in the current academic study of religion, this is presently not in vogue, but it has been endorsed to varying degrees by many influential religious scholars, including William James, Rudolf Otto, Aldous Huxley, Ninian Smart, Huston Smith, and Robert Forman.

Over the centuries, Buddhism, like Christianity, has produced a rich diversity of ways of viewing ultimate reality, the phenomenal world, and human nature. But there may be a luminous common ground in their deepest contemplative insights that is temporarily veiled by the biases and obscurations of the human mind. As William James commented, mystical states "offer us *hypotheses*, hypotheses which we may voluntarily ignore, but which as thinkers we cannot possibly upset. The supernaturalism and optimism to which they would persuade us may, interpreted in one way or another, be after all the truest of insights into the meaning of this life."[44]

6

WORLDS OF INTERSUBJECTIVITY

INTERSUBJECTIVITY LIES AT the very heart of the Buddhist world-view and its path to spiritual awakening. According to this theory, each person exists as an individual, but the self, or personal identity, is not an independent ego that is somehow in control of the body and mind. Rather, the individual is understood as a matrix of dependently related events in a state of flux. There are three aspects to this dependence: 1) the self arises in dependence upon prior contributing causes and conditions, such as parents and all others who contribute to one's survival, education, and so on. In this way, our existence is invariably intersubjective, for we exist in a causal nexus in which we are constantly influenced by and exert influence upon the world around us, including other people; 2) the individual self does not exist independently of the body and mind, but rather in reliance upon myriad physical and mental processes that are constantly changing; 3) according to the Middle Way view, which seeks to avoid the two extremes of substantialism and nihilism, the self is brought into existence by the power of conceptual imputation. That is, on the basis of either some aspect of the body (e.g., I am tall) or some mental process (e.g., I am content), the self is conceptually imputed *upon something it is not*. Thus, even though I am not the height of my body or the affective state of being content, within the conceptual framework in which I think of myself and others think of me, it is conventionally valid to assert that I am tall and content.

Moreover, Buddhism maintains that conceptual frameworks are not private; they are public and consensual. So the ways I perceive and conceive of myself and others are inextricably related to the community of language of users and thinkers with whom I share a common language and conceptual framework. We view ourselves, others, and the world around us by way of shared ideas, without which the world *as we perceive it and conceive of it* would not exist. Thus, our very existence as individuals, whether living in a community or in solitude, is intersubjective to the core.

What are the ramifications of this way of viewing reality? Here I shall focus on the following five questions, all pertaining closely to the idea of intersubjectivity:

1. Does individual human consciousness emerge solely from the dynamic interrelation of self and other, making it therefore inherently intersubjective? I shall address this topic within the framework of the Buddhist practice of the cultivation of meditative quiescence (*śamatha*), in which the conceptual mind is stilled and the attention is withdrawn away from the physical senses and purely into the realm of mental consciousness.

2. In what ways does Buddhist meditation cultivate a sense of empathy as an indispensable means for gaining insight into the nature of oneself, others, and the relation between oneself and the rest of the world? The response will be presented in accordance with the central Buddhist insight practice of the "four applications of mindfulness," in which one attends to the nature of the body, feelings, mental processes, and mental objects.

3. How does the theme of intersubjectivity pertain to Buddhist practices designed to induce greater empathy with others? In response to this question, I shall explain the Buddhist cultivation of the "four immeasurables," namely, loving-kindness, compassion, empathetic joy, and equanimity.

4. What significance does the Buddhist emphasis on the dreamlike nature of waking reality have for the issue of intersubjectivity? Here I will focus on the meditative practice of "dream yoga," which begins with training to induce lucid dreaming, or apprehending the dream state for what it is while dreaming.

5. Finally, how does Buddhism challenge the assertion of the existence of an inherently real, localized, ego-centered mind, and in what ways does it challenge the dichotomy of objective space and perceptual space? I will explain some of the essentials of the theory and practice of the Great Perfection tradition of Tibetan Buddhism, aimed at fathoming the essential nature of awareness.[1]

MEDITATIVE QUIESCENCE

In Buddhism, the development of meditative quiescence is regarded as an indispensable prerequisite for the cultivation of contemplative insight. The fundamental distinction between the two disciplines is that the practice of quiescence involves refining the attention by means of enhancing attentional stability and vividness and counteracting the mind's habitual tendencies toward alternating attentional excitation and laxity. The cultivation of contemplative insight, on the other hand, entails the precise examination and investigation of various facets of reality, using the previously refined attentional abilities. Thus, the training in quiescence may be regarded as a kind of contemplative technology, aimed at developing one of the primary tools by means of which mental phenomena can be directly explored. The training in insight may be viewed as a kind of contemplative science, aimed at acquiring experiential knowledge of the mind, the phenomena that are apprehended by it, and the relation between the two.[2]

Buddhism asserts that human beings with unimpaired sense faculties have six modes of perception. Five of those modes are by way of the five physical senses, and the sixth is mental perception, by means of which we perceive mental phenomena, such as thoughts, mental imagery, dreams, and emotions. Mental perception is viewed as being quite distinct from our capacity to think, remember, and imagine, all of which are conceptual faculties. Among the six modes of perception, the five physical senses can, at least in principle, be corrected, enhanced, and extended by external, technological means. Common examples in the modern world (though not in classical India or Tibet) are the use of eyeglasses to correct vision and the use of telescopes and microscopes to enhance and extend our visual capacities.

Mental perception is not readily amenable to technological enhancement, but among the six senses it is, according to Buddhism, the one that can be the most refined and extended through training. To start with, the normal untrained mind, which is so prone to alternating bouts of compulsive excitation and laxity, is regarded as "dysfunctional." So the bad news is that most of us are "attentionally challenged," regardless of whether we suffer from attention deficit (laxity) or hyperactivity (excitation) disorders. But the good news is that this mental disability can be successfully treated with rigorous, sustained training.

Traditionally, Buddhists who are dedicated to exploring the extent to which attentional stability and vividness can be enhanced are advised to disengage temporarily from social activity. Withdrawing into solitude for a period of weeks, months, or even years, they radically simplify their lifestyle and devote themselves single-pointedly to training the attention, while remaining as free as possible from all distracting influences. As long as we are actively engaged in society, our sense of personal identity is strongly reinforced by our intersubjective relations with others. But through withdrawal into solitude, our identity is significantly decontextualized. Externally, by disengaging from social interactions, the sense of self as holding a position in society is eroded. Internally, by disengaging from ideation—such as conceptually dwelling on events from our personal history, thinking about ourselves in the present, and anticipating what we will do in the future—our sense of self as occupying a real place in nature is eroded. To be decontextualized is to be deconstructed. This is one reason why in traditional societies, being sent into exile was regarded as one of the most severe forms of punishment, almost as drastic as capital punishment. And in the penal systems of modern society, one of the most severe forms of punishment is solitary confinement.

This existential shift is not undertaken casually or without suitable preparation. To illustrate this point, the Buddha gave the analogy of a great elephant that enters a shallow pond in order to enjoy the pleasures of drinking and bathing.[3] Due to its great size, the elephant finds footing in the deep water and enjoys itself thoroughly. But when a cat seeks to emulate the elephant by jumping into the pond, it finds no footing and either sinks or thrashes around on the surface. Here is the meaning of this parable. If one is inadequately prepared for the austere simplicity of the reclusive life, while dwelling for a sustained period in solitude, the mind either sinks by way of laxity into dullness, boredom, and depression, or else rises by way of excitation into compulsive ideation and sensory distractions. The critical issue is whether one has cultivated sufficient emotional stability and balance to be able to live happily without reliance upon the hedonic pleasures aroused by agreeable sensual, intellectual, aesthetic, and interpersonal stimuli. The single most powerful practice for achieving such emotional health is the cultivation of a sense of connectedness with others. This is done by empathetically reflecting again and again on others as subjects like oneself, with their hopes and fears, joys and sorrows, successes and failures. In this way, whether alone or with others, one overcomes the sense of loneliness and isolation.

Among the many techniques taught in Buddhism for training the attention, the most widely practiced entails cultivating mindfulness of the breathing. One begins by focusing the attention on the tactile sensations of the breath at the apertures of the nostrils. Over time, the body comes to feel light, and the respiration becomes more and more subtle. Eventually, while focusing the attention on the point of contact of the breath, right there a mental image spontaneously arises, on which one then sustains the attention. The type of image that arises varies from one person to the next, but may appear, for example, like a star, a round ruby, or a pearl.[4] This mental object remains the focus of attention until eventually it is replaced by a far subtler "counterpart sign," which also may arise in a variety of forms.

At this point, the attention is so concentrated in the field of mental perception that the mind is free of all physical sense impressions, including those of the body. If one then disengages the attention from the counterpart sign without relinquishing the heightened sense of attentional stability and vividness, in this absence of appearances comes the experience of a primal state of contentless awareness, the *bhavaṅga*, or "ground of becoming," from which all active mental processes arise.[5] As mentioned previously, this mode of awareness is said to shine with its own radiance, which is obscured only due to internal and external stimuli; and it is experienced as being primordially pure, regardless of whether it is temporarily blocked by adventitious defilements.[6] Remarkably, some Buddhist contemplatives have also found that the nature of this relative ground state of consciousness is loving-kindness, and it is regarded as the source of people's incentive to meditatively develop their minds in the pursuit of spiritual liberation.[7]

The experience of such a state of contentless mental awareness is common to various schools of Indian and Tibetan Buddhist meditation, as well as other, non-Buddhist contemplative traditions.[8] So there are empirical grounds for concluding that this is not simply a matter of speculation but rather an element of experience for contemplatives trained in a variety of techniques and adhering to a wide range of philosophical beliefs. If so, the possibility of such experience has profound implications for questions concerning the nature of consciousness. Is consciousness essentially intersubjective in the sense that its very nature, with its own innate luminosity, emerges by the relation of the self to others? The observation that the *bhavaṅga* is of the nature of love implies that empathy is innate to consciousness and exists prior to the emergence of all active mental processes. This, in turn, implies that empathy on the part of researchers must be a prerequisite for any genuine science of consciousness. On the other hand, the assertion that this state of awareness is free of all sensory and mental appearances implies a degree of autonomy from language, conceptual frameworks, and active engagement with others. So consciousness is not really *constituted* by the relation of the self to others, but rather is intersubjective in the weaker sense of simply being inherently open to and connected with others—an important theme to which I will return.

THE FOUR APPLICATIONS OF MINDFULNESS

The cultivation of compassion is like a silken thread that runs through and connects all the pearls of Buddhist meditative practices. Compassion is based upon empathy, but in a very deep sense, insight into the nature of oneself, others, and the relation between oneself and the rest of the world is also synergistically related to empathy. Moreover, a common Buddhist adage states that compassion without wisdom is bondage, and wisdom without compassion is another form of bondage. Thus, these qualities must be cultivated together, and empathy is a common root of both.

The classic Buddhist system of meditative practices known as the four applications of mindfulness is based on the *Satipaṭṭhānasutta*, the most revered of all Buddhist discourses in the Theravāda tradition.[9] This practice entails the careful observation and consideration of the body, feelings, mental processes, and mental objects of oneself and of others. A common theme within each of these four applications of mindfulness is first considering these elements of one's own being, then attending to the same phenomena in others, and finally shifting attention back and forth between self and others. Especially in the final phase of practice, one engages in what has recently been called "reiterated empathy," imaginatively viewing one's own psychophysical processes from a "second-person" perspective. That is, I view my body and mind from what I imagine to be your perspective, so that I begin to sense my own presence not only "from within" but "from without." Such practice leads to the insight that the second-person perspective on one's own being is just as "real" as the first-person perspective, and neither exists independently of the other.

Another of the central aims of these four applications of mindfulness is to distinguish between the phenomena that are presented to our six modes of perception and the conceptual superimpositions that we often unconsciously and involuntarily place upon them, including labels, categories, and thoughts aroused by emotional reactions. The Buddha summed up this theme when he declared, "In the seen there is only the seen; in the heard, there is only the heard; in the sensed, there is only the sensed; in the cognized, there is only the cognized."[10] Such practice leads to a kind of objectivity, perceiving things to a greater extent as they are, prior to personal conceptual overlays, judgments, and evaluations.

The first subject for the close application of mindfulness is the body, for this is our physical basis in reality, on which we most readily identify our whereabouts and distinguish ourselves from others. The Buddha quintessentially describes this practice as follows: "One dwells observing the body as the body internally, or one dwells observing the body as the body externally, or one dwells observing the body as the body both internally and externally."[11] In Pāli the term translated here as "observing" (*anupassati*) has the various meanings of "observing," "contemplating," and "considering," which override any strict demarcation between pure perception and conceptual reflection. It means taking in the observed phenomena as fully as possible, both perceptually and conceptually, while still being sensitive to practical distinctions between what is presented to the senses and what is superimposed upon them. So it has a considerably richer connotation than "bare attention," in the sense of moment-to-moment, nonjudgmental awareness of whatever arises. Such practice is done not only while sitting quietly in meditation but also while engaging in the various postures of walking, standing, sitting, and lying down, as well as the activities of looking, bending, stretching, dressing, eating, drinking, excreting, speaking, keeping silent, staying awake, and falling asleep.[12]

While first attending to one's own body, one observes, among other things, the various events or factors that give rise to the emergence and dissolution of experiences of and in the body. By *observing* rather than simply *identifying* with it, the body is experienced simply as a network of phenomena, rather than as a self. Then, on the basis of the experiential insights gained in this way, one perceptually observes the body of another, experiencing that also as a matrix of phenomena. Finally, one alternates between observing both one's own body and another's body, perceiving qualities that are unique to each as well as common characteristics, which might include events that lead to the emergence and dissolution of body events from moment to moment.

The most important common characteristic of bodies is that none of them either is or contains a self, or personal identity. They are simply phenomena, arising in dependence upon prior causes and conditions. Realizing this begins to break down the reified sense of the locality of one's presence as being solely within the confines of one's own body. As William James declares, phenomenologically speaking, *"for the moment, what we attend to is reality."*[13] By habitually failing to attend either to one's own body or those of others, the bodies that we disregard are eventually not counted as existing. As James comments, "They are not even treated as appearances; they are treated as if they were mere waste, equivalent to nothing at all."[14] Moreover, by attending internally, externally, and finally internally and externally in immediate succession, one neutralizes any biases of attention that might result from one's own introverted or extroverted disposition. In addition, this final phase of alternating the attention between self and others affords the opportunity to observe relationships that may not be apparent as long as one is focused on the self to the exclusion of others. And as James cogently argues, very much in accordance with Buddhist principles, *"The relations that connect experi-*

ences must themselves be experienced relations, and any kind of relation experienced must be accounted as 'real' as anything else in the system."[15]

In the traditional practice of applying mindfulness to feelings, one observes the arising and dissolution of the three basic kinds of feelings of physical and mental pleasure, pain, and indifference in oneself, others, and alternately between oneself and others. Other, more complex affective states are left to the next level of practice, but special attention is given to pleasant and unpleasant feelings because these have such an enormous effect on the kinds of choices we make and the ways we lead our lives.

While classical cognitive science has been "cognocentric," in the sense of maintaining that humans are cognizers first and foremost, recent advances in affective psychology and neuroscience suggest that emotions are primary, and cognition has a secondary role as an organizing influence. According to Buddhism, neither cognition nor emotion is primary; rather, they are co-emergent, incapable of existing without the other. It is important to bear in mind, however, that the feeling of indifference, which some might regard as being an *absence* of feeling, is regarded in Buddhism as also being an affective state.

When observing the arising, presence, and dissolution of feelings firsthand, one recognizes that they are experienced in various regions throughout the body, and some do not appear to have any identifiable location at all. When empathetically attending to others' joys and sorrows, pleasures and pains, one may ask: Are such "observations" of others' internal affective states strictly inferential? That is, are these observations really conceptual conclusions based upon perceived outward signs? Or might this type of empathetic awareness be more direct, more akin to perception? I am not aware that either Buddhism or modern science has reached a consensus regarding these questions, but I believe they merit careful consideration.

The cultivation of mindfulness of mental processes follows the threefold sequence as above, while observing the mind as it is affected by different conative, attentional, cognitive, and affective states, such as craving, hatred, delusion, anxiety, elation, concentration, and agitation. The aim of this practice is explicitly therapeutic in nature. Some conative, attentional, cognitive, and affective states and processes are conducive to one's own and others' well-being; others are harmful. By attending closely to the factors that give rise to a wide range of mental processes and by observing the effects they have on self and others, one begins to recognize through experience those processes that are conducive to one's own and others' well-being and those that are destructive. In this way one identifies the distinctions between wholesome and unwholesome mental states. This is an essential element of mindfulness within Buddhist practice. As one authoritative Theravāda text declares, "Mindfulness, when it arises, follows the courses of beneficial and unbeneficial tendencies, [recognizing] these tendencies are beneficial, these unbeneficial; these tendencies are helpful, these unhelpful. Thus, one who practices yoga rejects unbeneficial tendencies and cultivates beneficial tendencies."[16]

In particular, like a physician diagnosing an illness, one pays special attention to what Buddhism calls "mental afflictions," which can be identified by the criterion that they disrupt the balance and equilibrium of the mind. While some wholesome mental processes, such as compassion, may indeed disturb the calm of the mind, this disruption is not deep, and its long-term effects on mental states and behavior are healthy. Other processes, however, such as resentment, have a deep and harmful impact on mental health as well as subsequent behavior, so they are deemed afflictions.

As in the previous practices of attending mindfully to the body and feelings, in this phase of the practice one observes one's own and others' mental processes simply as impersonal phenomena, arising in dependence upon prior causes and conditions, paying special attention to the duration of these mental states: how long does each one last, and for as long as it lasts, does it exist as a stable entity persisting through time or as a sequence of momentary events? When one observes a process in one's own mental continuum, is it affected by the sheer fact of being observed? Is it possible to observe a mental state with an awareness that is not itself in that same state? For example, is it possible to observe anger with a calm, dispassionate awareness? Does one observe an intentional mental process *while* it is occurring, or is such mindfulness always retrospective? It is important to bear in mind that the Pāli term commonly translated as "mindfulness" (*sati*) also has the connotation of "recollection," implying that many, if not all, acts of mindfulness may actually be modes of short-term recall. The issue of observer participancy is obviously crucial to the first-person examination of mental states, and it should by no means disqualify such introspective inquiry any more than it has disqualified exploration in the field of quantum mechanics.

The fourth phase of this practice is the cultivation of mindfulness of mental objects, which include all nonintentional mental processes as well as all other kinds of phenomena that can be apprehended with the mind. Thus, this category is all-inclusive. At the same time, there is a special emphasis on observing in oneself, others, and both oneself and others the contents of the mind affiliated with wholesome and unwholesome mental states, as well as the conditions leading to their emergence and dissolution. In addition, one mindfully observes all the phenomena of the environment from one's own perspective by means of direct perception and empathetically attends to them from the perspective of others. The overarching theme of all these practices is the cultivation of a multiperspectival view of the self, others, and the intersubjective relations between them. The techniques are explicitly designed to yield insights into these facets of the lived world, but they all have a strong bearing on the cultivation of compassion and other wholesome affective states, without which the cultivation of wisdom alone is said to be one more form of bondage.

THE FOUR IMMEASURABLES

Just as the qualities of cognizance and loving-kindness are coexistent in the ground state of awareness known as the *bhavaṅga*, so too in the course of spiritual maturation must the light of insight and the warmth of a loving heart be cultivated together. Therefore, in Buddhism the four applications of mindfulness are traditionally complemented by the cultivation of the four immeasurables, namely loving-kindness, compassion, empathetic joy, and equanimity.[17]

Each of these affective states can easily be conflated with other emotions that may appear similar but are fundamentally different. To help distinguish between the affective states to be cultivated and their false facsimiles, it may be helpful to draw on the classification of different types of relations proposed by the philosopher Martin Buber in his classic work *I and Thou*.[18] We can begin with what Buber calls an "I-it" relationship, in which one engages with another sentient being viewed simply as an object, to be manipulated in accordance with one's self-centered desires. In such a relationship the other's existence as a subject fundamentally like oneself is ignored or marginalized, viewed only in terms of how he or she (really "it") may be of aid, be an obstacle, or be irrelevant in the pursuit of one's own goals. On that basis, this individual comes to be regarded as a friend, enemy, or someone of no consequence. In an "I-it" relationship there is effectively only one subject, oneself, but in explicitly dehumanizing the other, one is implicitly dehumanizing oneself as well.

An "I-you" relationship, on the other hand, is essentially dialogical in the sense of one subject meaningfully engaging with the subjective reality of another person. While an "I-it" relationship is fundamentally manipulative, an "I-you" relationship is intersubjective and therefore based upon a sense of empathy. According to Buber, in the midst of an "I-you" relationship, one may transcend the polarity of self and other and engage with a sphere between self and other, in which both access the "eternal thou" that transcends individuality. This cannot happen unless *both* subjects are involved in an "I-you" relationship. It is at heart a participatory experience.

Western thought, inspired by the Judeo-Christian and Greco-Roman traditions, is largely anthropocentric when it comes to intersubjective relationships. But according to Buddhism, all sentient beings strive to experience pleasure and joy and to avoid pain and suffering. This is an indication that Buddhism is rightly characterized as more biocentric than anthropocentric, and its aim is to cultivate loving-kindness and the other wholesome affective states in this tetrad for all sentient beings to a degree that transcends all boundaries and demarcations.

The first of the four states to be cultivated is loving-kindness, which is understood as the heartfelt yearning for the well-being of others. Although it is tempting to translate the corresponding Sanskrit term (*maitri*) simply as "love," it is not commonly done because in English, this term is often used in ways that conflate an "I-you" relationship with an "I-it" relationship. The loving-kindness cultivated in Buddhist practice emphatically entails an "I-you" relationship, for one is vividly aware of the other person's joys and sorrows, hopes and fears. But in English the word "love" is also used in cases of sexual infatuation, personal attachment, and even strong attraction to inanimate objects and events, all of which involve "I-it" relationships. In Buddhism an entirely different term (*rāga*) is generally used to denote such kinds of attraction, and it is variously translated as "attachment," "craving," or "obsession."

According to Buddhism, attachment is an attraction to an object on which one conceptually superimposes or exaggerates desirable qualities, while filtering out undesirable qualities. In cases of strong attachment, one transfers the very possibility of happiness onto the object, thereby disempowering oneself and empowering it. Even when such attachment is directed toward another person, it entails more of an "intrasubjective" than an intersubjective relationship, for one is engaging more poignantly with one's own conceptual superimpositions than with the other person as a genuine subject. When the reality of the idealized object of attachment—with all his or her faults and limitations—breaks through the fantasies, disillusionment may ensue. That in turn may lead to hostility and aversion, which superimposes negative qualities upon the person previously held dear.

Thus, according to Buddhism, loving-kindness does not readily turn into aversion, but attachment does. And while loving-kindness is a wholesome conative state (not simply an emotion) that is conducive to one's own and others' well-being, attachment is a major source of anxiety, distress, and interpersonal conflict. It is therefore very important not to conflate them, but in most close human relations, such as between parents and children, spouses, and friends, they are normally mixed. In these complex human relationships the Buddhist ideal is to attenuate the mental affliction of attachment and cultivate the wholesome conative state of loving-kindness.

In what may appear at first glance to be paradoxical, in traditional Buddhist practice one first cultivates loving-kindness for oneself, then proceeds to extend this affectionate concern to others. The rationale for this is based on a fundamental premise expressed by the Buddha, "Whoever loves himself will never harm another."[19] This strategy seems especially appropriate in the modern West, where feelings of self-contempt, low self-esteem, guilt, and being unworthy of happiness seem to have reached epidemic proportions.[20] In the meditative practice itself, one first attends to one's own longing for happiness and wish to be free of suffering, and generates the loving wish, "May I be free of animosity, affliction, and anxiety, and live happily." Like the preceding practices of mindfulness, this involves a process of objectifying oneself and yearning for the person brought to mind, "May you be well and happy." In this way one enters into an "I–you" relationship with oneself!

In the next phase of the practice, one brings to mind someone else whom one dearly loves and respects. Recalling this person's acts of kindness and virtues, one brings forth the heartfelt wish, "May this good person, like myself, be well and happy." Continuing in this practice, one similarly brings to mind in sequence a more casual friend, then a person toward whom one has been indifferent, and finally a person toward whom one has felt aversion. The aim of the practice is to gradually experience the same degree of loving-kindness for the dear friend as for oneself, for the neutral person as for the dear friend, and finally for the enemy as for the neutral person. In this way, the conceptually superimposed "I–it" barriers demarcating friend, stranger, and foe are broken down, and immeasurable, unconditional loving-kindness may be experienced.

As stated previously, the false facsimile of loving-kindness is attachment. According to Buddhism, the opposite of loving-kindness is not indifference but hatred. While indifference may be viewed as being turned 90 degrees away from loving-kindness, hatred is turned 180 degrees away, for when the mind is dominated by hatred, one actually feels *unhappy* at the prospect of another's well-being. The proximate cause of loving-kindness is seeing loveable qualities within others, not merely their outer, surface attractions. One succeeds in this practice when it causes animosity to subside, and fails when it leads only to selfish affection, or attachment, for this implies that one is still stuck in an "I–it" mentality.

The second of the four immeasurables is compassion, which is inextricably linked with loving-kindness. With loving-kindness one yearns that others may find genuine happiness and the causes of happiness, and with compassion one yearns that they may be free of suffering and its causes. These are really two sides of the same coin. While attachment is frequently confused with loving-kindness, righteous indignation for the sake of others can easily be confused with compassion. If one's "compassion" extends only to the victims of the world and not to the victimizers, it is likely to be another case of attachment to the downtrodden, combined with aversion to the oppressors. In other words, one is still trapped in an "I–it" mentality. The compassion cultivated in Buddhist practice is focused not only on those who are experiencing suffering and pain but also on those who are sowing the seeds of further suffering and pain (for themselves and others), namely those who maliciously harm others. According to Buddhism, all the evil in the world stems from attachment, aversion, and the delusion that underlies both. These destructive tendencies are regarded as mental afflictions, very much like physical afflictions, and those who are dominated by them are even more deserving of compassion than those afflicted with physical diseases. But to feel compassion for evildoers is not to condone the evil they commit. It is to yearn that they be free of the impulses that compel them to behave in such harmful ways, and thereby be free of the causes of suffering.

In the meditative cultivation of compassion, one attends first to someone who is wretched and miserable, wishing, "If only this person could be freed from such suffering!" Progressing in this practice, one then sequentially focuses on an evildoer (regardless of whether he or she seems happy), on a dear person, on a neutral person, and finally on someone toward whom one has felt aversion. The goal of the practice is like that of the cultivation of loving-kindness, namely, to break down the barriers separating the different types of individuals until one's compassion extends equally to all beings.

The false facsimile of compassion is grief. In English, compassion is often verbally expressed with a comment such as "I feel so sorry for that person," but according to Buddhism, merely feeling sympathy for someone does not necessarily include compassion. When one empathetically attends to another person who is unhappy, one naturally experiences sadness. But such a feeling may lead instead to righteous indignation and the vengeful wish to exact retribution on whoever has made the other person unhappy. On the other hand, in the cultivation of compassion, sympathy acts instead as fuel for the warmth of compassion. One does not simply remain in a state of sadness or despair, but rises from it with the wish, "May you be free of this suffering and its causes!"—psychologically moving from the reality of the present suffering to the possibility of freedom from it.

The opposite of compassion is not indifference, but cruelty. When this mental affliction dominates the mind, one insidiously acknowledges the subjective reality of the other and wishes for that person to experience misery. This is widely regarded as the greatest evil to which the mind can succumb. The proximate cause of compassion is seeing the helplessness in those overwhelmed by suffering and its causes, while also recognizing the possibility of freedom from such misery. One succeeds in this practice when one's own proneness to cruelty subsides, and fails when the practice produces only sorrow. It is important to emphasize that the Buddhist meditative cultivation of loving-kindness and compassion was never intended as a *substitute* for active service to others. Rather, it is a *mental preparation* for such altruistic service that raises the likelihood of such outer behavior being truly an expression of an inner, benevolent concern for others' well-being.

The cultivation of the final two immeasurables follows naturally from progress in the cultivation of the first two. If one feels loving-kindness and compassion for others, then when they experience joy, the spontaneous response is to take delight in their happiness. But such empathetic joy can also be cultivated in its own right. In Buddhist practice, one focuses first on a very dear companion who is constantly of good cheer, then on a neutral person, and finally on a person who has shown hostility. In each case, one empathizes with the other's joy and experiences it as if it were one's own. However, it is possible get caught up in a kind of hedonistic pleasure in relation to others, which is the false facsimile of empathetic joy. The opposite of this wholesome affective state is envy; its proximate cause is the awareness of others' happiness and success; and one fails in this practice when it results in hedonism.

Equanimity, the fourth of the immeasurables, actually suffuses the other three, as the practitioner breaks down the self-centered divisions that are superimposed on other people. With equanimity, loving and compassionate concern for others extends out evenly, with no bias for friends or against enemies. Such equanimity is based upon empathy, recognizing that all beings, like oneself, are equally worthy of happiness. This meditative practice begins by focusing on a neutral person, then a dear person, and finally a hostile person, in each case resting in a state of equanimity free of attachment and aversion. The false facsimile of the equanimity to be cultivated here is stupid indifference, wherein one does not care about the well-being of anyone else. The opposite of equanimity is attachment to loved ones and aversion to enemies, and its proximate cause is said to be taking responsibility for one's own conduct. One succeeds in this practice when it produces equanimity that is a fertile, level ground for the growth of loving-kindness and compassion, and fails when it produces aloof indifference.

THE FOUR IMMEASURABLES

IMMEASURABLE	LOVING-KINDNESS	COMPASSION	EMPATHETIC JOY	EQUANIMITY
Proximate Cause	perceiving the loveableness of sentient beings	perceiving the helplessness of sentient beings	perceiving the joys and virtues of others	perceiving the responsibility for one's deeds
False Facsimile	self-centered attachment	grief	hedonic pleasure	aloof indifference
Opposite	malice	cruelty	envy	attachment and aversion
Sign of Success	animosity subsides	cruelty subsides	cynicism subsides	attachment and aversion subside
Sign of Failure	selfish affection arises	sorrow arises	frivolity arises	cold indifference arises

In the Tibetan Buddhist tradition, the cultivation of loving-kindness and compassion is combined in a classic practice known in Tibetan as *tonglen*, meaning "giving and taking."[21] The enactment of loving-kindness is the "giving" component of the practice, and the enactment of compassion is the "taking" component. The latter begins by bringing vividly to mind a loved one or a community of people or other beings who are either suffering or sowing the seeds of suffering by means of harmful conduct. First, through empathy, one enters into the suffering and the sources of suffering of this person, then generates the wish, "May you be relieved of this burden and may this adversity ripen upon me." Whatever the affliction or adversity, physical or mental, one imagines taking it upon oneself in the form of a black cloud being re-moved from the other's body and mind and drawn into one's heart. Simulta-neously, one imagines that the other person is gradually relieved of the bur-den. As soon as this dark cloud enters the heart, one imagines that it meets with the sense of self-centeredness, visualized as an orb of darkness. And in an instant, that cloud of misery and the darkness of one's self-centeredness extinguish each other, leaving not a trace of either behind.

In the "giving" component of this practice, one imagines all the prosper-ity, happiness, and goodness in one's life as a powerful wellspring of brilliant white light emanating from one's heart, reaching out and suffusing the other person as one wishes, "All that is good in my life, my possessions, my happi-ness, my good health, my virtues, I offer to you. May you be well and happy." One imagines the light of this virtue and happiness suffusing the person who has been brought to mind, and imagines his or her most meaningful desires and aspirations being fulfilled. Yet as this light from the heart flows forth unimpeded, it is not depleted, for it is imagined as arising from an inexhaust-ible source.

As familiarity is acquired with this meditative practice, one may expand the scope of awareness finally to include all sentient beings, taking in all suf-fering and mental afflictions and sending forth all one's virtue and goodness. This practice may then be conjoined with the breath: during each inhalation, one imagines taking in the burden of suffering and the sources of suffering, and with each exhalation rays of white light emerge from the heart, bringing happiness and the causes of happiness to all the world.

Śāntideva, on whose writings this practice is based, summed up the ratio-nale behind it: "I should eliminate the suffering of others because it is suf-fering, just like my own suffering. I should take care of others because they are sentient beings, just as I am a sentient being."[22] This is a pure expression of an "I–you" relationship with all sentient beings. The "I–thou" relationship as it is cultivated in Buddhist practice will be discussed in the next section.

DREAM YOGA

The word "buddha" means "one who is awake," and the implication is that everyone who is not a buddha is asleep, most of us leading lives very much akin to a nonlucid dream. According to the Middle Way view, mentioned at the beginning of this chapter, waking experience has a dreamlike quality because of the disparity between the way things appear and the way they exist. All phenomena—oneself, others, and everything else in the perceived environment—*appear* as if they bear their own inherent existence, independently of the conceptual frameworks within which they are apprehended. But in terms of the way they *exist*, all conditioned phenomena are dependent upon the causes and conditions that gave rise to them, their own parts and attributes, and the conceptual designations by which they are demarcated from other phenomena and by which they bear their own components and qualities. In short, oneself, other beings, and all other phenomena appear to exist in and of themselves, but nothing has such an independent existence. According to the Middle Way view, that very absence of an inherent identity of any phenomenon is called "emptiness."[23]

Tsongkhapa asserts, "Although the objects of perception have forever utterly lacked a final self-nature or objective existence, nonetheless they indisputably appear with the nature of having real, inherent existence.... These things function conventionally on the basis of the laws of interdependence and causality."[24] According to this view, the objects of perception—colors, sounds, smells, and so forth—do not exist in the objective world, independently of the sense modalities by which they are perceived. But, for example, do trees exist apart from our perception of them? The Middle Way answer is that trees and the many other objects in the natural world do indeed exist independently of our perceptions. Flowers continue to grow and bloom when no one is looking, and trees fall to the forest floor, sending out ripples in the atmosphere and over the ground, and then begin to decay, whether or not anyone is there to witness these events.

One may then ask, "Do flowers, trees, and other natural phenomena exist independently of any conceptual designations of them?" The answer is that the words "flowers," "trees," and so on have no meaning apart from the definitions we have attributed to them. Thus, the question has no meaning.[25] But we may then push this point and ask, "Does *anything* exist independently of human language and thought?" The question implies that the word "exist" is somehow self-defining, that it stands on its own, independent of any consensually accepted definition. But all terms such as "subject," "object," "existence," "reference," "meaning," "reason," "knowledge," "observation," and "experience" have a multitude of different uses, and none has a single absolute meaning to which priority must be granted. Since these terms are not self-defining, we employ their definitions according to the conceptual schemes of our choice. That is, we choose our definitions; they are not determined by objective reality. So, once again, proponents of the Middle Way view conclude that the question is meaningless: if the word "exist" has no meaning independent of all conceptual frameworks, then it makes no sense to ask whether anything exists independent of all conceptual frameworks.

For this reason the Middle Way view rejects metaphysical realism, which has been defined as the view that the world consists of mind-independent objects; there is exactly one true and complete description of the way the world is; and truth involves some sort of correspondence between an independently existent world and a description of it.[26] Scientists question nature with measuring devices created in collaboration with engineers. But the data collected arise in dependence upon both the objective phenomenon being studied and the measuring devices themselves. The data are thus produced as dependently related events, much as we hear sounds that are produced through the interaction of vibrations in some objective medium and our auditory faculties. But the *sounds we hear* do not exist *independently* in the objective world, nor do any of the other data collected by the instruments of technology.

Proponents of metaphysical realism might well grant this point but then counter that the conceptual world of physics exists, based upon objective magnitudes, and corresponds to the real, objective world, existing independent of language and thought. However, as scientists interpret the data gathered from their measuring devices, they must distinguish between significant data and "noise." Moreover, the theory they are using plays an instrumental role in such choices, just as it does in determining what types of measuring devices to create and how to interpret the data gathered from them. In all cases, what is finally "observed" is deeply theory-laden.

Thus, the perceptual objects detected with the senses or with the instruments of technology do not exist independent of those modes of detection, and they do not exist independent of the conceptual frameworks through which such measurements are filtered. Moreover, the theoretical entities conceived of by physicists are comprised of related events arising in dependence upon both observational data and the conceptual faculties of the scientists who interpret and make sense of those data. This implies the intersubjective nature of perceptual as well as conceptual experience, especially when we consider the consensual nature of conceptual frameworks.

While the Middle Way view has certain similarities with the thought of some of the founders of quantum theory, among contemporary philosophies it is perhaps most akin to the pragmatic realism of Hilary Putnam. In a statement closely in accord with the writings of Nāgārjuna, Putnam declares, "Elements of what we call 'language' or 'mind' *penetrate so deeply into what we call 'reality' that the very project of representing ourselves as being 'map-*

pers' of something 'language-independent' is fatally compromised from the very start."[27] If there were no language users, there would not be anything true or anything with sense or reference. Thus, the rich and ever-growing collection of truths about the world is the product of experience intertwined with language users, who play a creative role in producing our knowledge of the world.

According to the views of both the Middle Way and pragmatic realism, once we have chosen a conceptual scheme, there are facts to be discovered, not merely legislated by our language or concepts. Our conceptual scheme restricts the range of descriptions available to us, but it does not predetermine the answers to our questions. In accordance with the Middle Way view, Putnam writes, "The stars are indeed independent of our minds in the sense of being causally independent; we did not make the stars.... The fact that there is no one metaphysically privileged description of the universe does not mean that the universe depends on our minds."[28]

While the Middle Way view rejects the philosophical extreme of metaphysical realism, it equally rejects the cultural relativist or postmodernist view that no truth claims can be made in ways that transcend the culture in which they are embedded. For example, the assertion that all phenomena are empty of inherent existence is regarded as a universal truth, not contingent upon the beliefs of any one person or society. The Buddhist laws of karma are also presented as truths that are independent of any specific culture, time, or place. The Middle Way view also rejects materialism and philosophical idealism as two metaphysical extremes, each reifying the phenomenon of its choice—matter or mind—as being inherently real, independent of conceptual designation.

The Middle Way view provides the philosophical framework for the contemplative practice of dream yoga. In a nonlucid dream—in which there is no recognition that one is dreaming—all objective phenomena seem to exist in and of themselves. They, like one's own persona in the dream, seem to be real. But upon waking, one recognizes that neither one's own mind nor any person or situation encountered in the dream had any such independent existence. This is equally true during the waking state, and in the daytime practice of dream yoga, one maintains this awareness as constantly as possible. Everything experienced throughout the day—contrary to appearances—arises in relation to one's own perceptions and conceptions. Every person encountered is perceived and conceived in relation to one's own sensory and conceptual faculties. Never does one encounter the radically and absolutely "other," for apprehension of the other is always dependent upon one's own subjective perspective. Thus, upon fathoming the emptiness of inherent existence of all waking phenomena, one maintains throughout the day a sense of the dreamlike quality of all events, recognizing the profoundly intersubjective nature of all relationships with other beings and the environment.[29]

As in modern techniques for inducing lucid dreaming, the daytime practice of dream yoga is complemented with nighttime practices.[30] Although many specific methods are taught, one common to the modern techniques and to dream yoga is to fall asleep with the strong resolution to apprehend the dream state as such while actually dreaming. It can be difficult to recognize the dream for what it is and difficult to maintain that awareness without either waking up immediately or fading back into a nonlucid dream, but when success in this practice is achieved, it often comes with a sense of great freedom and exhilaration. One now knows that one's own body and everything else in the dream are manifestations of one's own substrate consciousness, and even with no sensory experience of the body lying in bed, one inferentially knows it is there, outside the context of the dream. In a nonlucid dream one has a very definite sense of one's own locality: other people in the dream are apprehended as being really "over there." But in a lucid dream, one is aware that everyone is an individual expression of some facet of the substrate consciousness.

To clarify this point: other people and objects in my dream are not manifestations of my mind as one more character in the dream; rather, they, like myself in the dream, are manifestations of my substrate consciousness, while I am asleep *outside* the dream. The dreamed self's mind still seems to be local, but in a lucid dream the dreamer is aware that his or her mind pervades all people, things, and events. So the lucid dreamer is, so to speak, localized as the dreamed persona, but nonlocalized in the knowledge of the self as being the dreamer. Another way of saying this is that as a dreamed persona, one engages in *intersubjective* relations with others in the dream, but with the recognition of oneself as the dreamer, one knows all these encounters to be *intrasubjective*. A lucid dreamer is aware of both these perspectives, and in the awareness that transcends the duality of self and others in the dream, enters into an "I–thou" relationship with the other, who is none other than the self.

This insight into nonduality enables one to see the fallacy of viewing others in the dream as being independently worthy of either hatred or attachment. If someone else in the dream has done something reprehensible, the agent of that act is not absolutely different from oneself and has no independent existence whatsoever. Likewise, if there is someone very attractive in the dream, out of habit, one may still experience desire, but know that the object of craving is a creation of one's own substrate consciousness. To overcome that habitual craving, one must thoroughly familiarize oneself with the insight that the object has no independent, objective existence.[31] When this insight penetrates waking experience as well, this opens up the possibility of cultivating an "I–thou" relationship with others throughout the course of one's life.

Particularly in a lucid dream, one has the sense of perceiving events in the "private theater" of the mind, but Buddhism nevertheless maintains that this theater is pervious to external, spatially and temporally nonlocal influences. For example, this tradition accepts the possibility of precognition and remote viewing occurring in a dream, as well as during the waking state. Given the possibility of outside influences impinging, the dreamscape may be likened to an open-air theater, in which one may not only perceive what is taking place on stage but also hear crickets from the surrounding fields and jets flying overhead. Likewise, during the waking state, the field of mental perception—that domain in which one experiences mental imagery while awake and dreams while asleep—is equally open to outside influences. This raises the fascinating question as to the whereabouts of the borders of the mind and how porous those borders are, if any can be found.

In the practice of dream yoga there are further techniques to be applied after one has apprehended the dream state for what it is, but here I shall focus on the practice of cultivating lucid dreamless sleep. Padmasambhava writes:[32]

> When you are fast asleep, if the vivid, indivisibly clear and empty light of deep sleep is recognized, the clear light is apprehended. One who remains without losing the experience of meditation all the time while asleep, without the advent of dreams or latent predispositions, is one who dwells in the nature of the clear light of sleep.

What he is describing is the nature of primordial consciousness when it is perceived devoid of content and conceptual structuring. This is called the "clear light" of awareness, about which Padmasambhava writes, "The nature of the clear light, even after the stream of thoughts has ceased and you have gone asleep, is a clear and empty phenomenon of the dream-state, which is like the center of limpid space, remaining nakedly, without an object."[33]

While the cultivation of meditative quiescence alone may withdraw the mind into the relative ground state of awareness, known as the substrate consciousness or ground of becoming, that does not ensure that one will actually ascertain the clear, empty, luminous nature of primordial consciousness. That is one of the goals of dream yoga, which is practiced while sleeping, and it is also the goal of the Great Perfection, which is primarily practiced while in the waking state.

THE GREAT PERFECTION

The theory and practice of the Great Perfection is based upon and perfectly compatible with the Middle Way view discussed earlier. The Great Perfection is considered by many Tibetans as the pinnacle of Buddhist insight, and it challenges the view that the human mind exists inherently independent of all conceptual frameworks. Cutting to the core of our very identity, the practice of the Great Perfection probes into the deeply held assumption that there is such a thing as an inherently real, localized, ego-centered mind.

The classic strategy for investigating the ontological status of the mind according to this tradition is to examine firsthand the mode of origination, the location, and the mode of dissolution of mental events, including awareness itself.[34] A primary challenge in this practice is to distinguish, by means of penetrating mindfulness, between what is perceptually given and what is conceptually superimposed upon perceptual experience. In this mode of contemplative inquiry, one focuses entirely on the *phenomena* of mental events, attending closely to the precise manner in which they arise in the field of mental perception. This contemplative inquiry is guided by such questions as, "Do they arise all at once or gradually? Can their place of origin be identified? What is the nature of that out of which these mental events arise?" In English, as in Sanskrit and Tibetan, it is often said that thoughts and emotions emerge from, or are produced by, the mind. One now seeks out the referent of "the mind" from which mental events allegedly arise.

In the second phase of this investigation, one attends closely to the location of mental events. Once again, one seeks to let *experience* answer this question, as opposed to preconceptions. Many neuroscientists claim that all mental events are located in the brain, and the basis for their assertion is the wide range of mind-brain correlates that they have ingeniously discovered. But the fact that two events, A and B, are temporally or causally correlated does not logically or empirically require that B is located in A or that A is located in B. Thus, the close correlations between mental and neural events no more require that the mental events be located in the neural events than they require that the neural events be located in the mental events. And the temporal or causal correlation of the two certainly does not necessitate the conclusion that they are equivalent!

Another recent scientific hypothesis is that mental processes are embodied in the sensorimotor activity of the organism and are embedded in the environment. In the practice of the Great Perfection one puts all such speculations to the experiential test by closely examining the location of mental events firsthand. This inquiry is led by questions such as, "Are mental events located in the body? If so, in exactly which part of the body are they experienced as being present? If they are found to exist outside the body, where in the environment are they specifically located? Does the awareness of mental events have the same location as those objects of awareness?" Mental events are commonly said to exist "in the mind," so in this practice one meticulously examines the nature of the perceptual space in which they purportedly take place. It is worth noting that such contemplative inquiry is commonly practiced while sitting motionless, so sensorimotor activity is held to a minimum. This has been found to facilitate attentional stability, but it certainly does not, by itself, decrease the amount of mental activity, which would be surprising if such activity were actually located in sensorimotor processes.

Finally, in this sequence of investigations, one examines how mental events disappear, whether gradually or suddenly, and inspects that into which they disappear. Some Buddhist writings suggest that they return to the substrate consciousness, where they are stored as propensities, or latent impulses. In this practice one is once again seeking out the real referent of the word "mind."

The essence of the Great Perfection practice of investigating the nature of the mind is stated succinctly by Padmasambhava:[35]

> While steadily maintaining the gaze, place the awareness unwaveringly, steadily, clearly, nakedly and fixedly without having anything on which to meditate in the sphere of space. When stability increases, examine the consciousness that is stable. Then gently release and relax. Again place it steadily and steadfastly observe the consciousness of that moment. What is the nature of that mind? Let it steadfastly observe itself. Is it something clear and steady or is it an emptiness that is nothing? Is there something there to recognize? Look again and report your experience to me!

By means of such inquiry, Buddhist contemplatives have come to the conclusion that the mind and awareness itself are not intrinsically identifiable. When sought out as inherently existing things or events, they are not to be found. This is equally true of all other perceptual and conceptual objects of awareness. The mind, like all other phenomena, is discovered to be empty, but it is not a mere vacuity. Rather, it is luminous, cognizant, and empty like boundless space, with no center or periphery, suffused with transparent light. Out of this luminous space of nonlocal awareness, all phenomena arise in relation to the conceptual frameworks within which they are designated. But neither the objects of awareness nor awareness itself can be said to exist independently of their conceptual designations. Recognition of this fundamental nature of the world of experience lends a dreamlike quality to life as a whole, in which all reified distinctions between subject and object, self and other, vanish.

Once one has recognized the lack of inherent existence of the mind and all mental objects, one is ready to be introduced to the nature of primordial consciousness that transcends all conceptual constructs, including the notions of existence and nonexistence. This is the central theme of practice of the Great Perfection and is considered the deepest of all insights. Padmasambhava points out the nature of primordial consciousness as follows:[36]

> To introduce this by pointing it out directly, past consciousness has disappeared without a trace. Moreover, future realization is unarisen, and in the freshness of its own present, unfabricated way of being, there is the ordinary consciousness of the present. When it peers into itself, with this observation there is a vividness in which nothing is seen. This awareness is direct, naked, vivid, unestablished, empty, limpid luminosity, unique, nondual clarity and emptiness. It is not permanent, but unestablished. It is not nihilistic, but radiantly vivid. It is not one, but is manifoldly aware and clear. It is not manifold, but is indivisibly of one taste. It is none other than this very self-awareness. This is an authentic introduction to the primordial nature of being.

In this intimate exchange between contemplative mentor and student, the mentor ideally speaks directly out of immediate experience of pure awareness, and by receiving this introduction, the student identifies his or her own primordial consciousness firsthand. Unlike in conventional modes of cognition, that which is apprehended and that which apprehends are identical. Such a mentor–student encounter is a paradigmatic "I–thou" relationship, in which both realize a nonlocal reality that transcends the individuation of the subjects. But the realization of primordial consciousness can also occur without engaging with another person. It does not arise from the interaction of two subjects, but rather transcends the distinctions among all subjects and objects.

In the practice of the Great Perfection, close attention is paid to the spaces in which physical and mental phenomena appear to originate, abide, and disappear. At the outset there seem to be two distinct kinds of space: external space, in which one experiences the environment, other people, and even one's own body, and internal space, in which one experiences one's own private mental processes, such as thoughts, emotions, mental imagery, and dreams. According to Buddhist theory as a whole, all outer, public events and all inner, private events are equally "natural," in the sense of arising in dependence upon prior causes and conditions. The notion that only matter and its properties are "natural," while anything immaterial is "unnatural" or "supernatural," is utterly alien to the Buddhist understanding of the world.

According to the Buddhist view, the natural world is filled with myriad phenomena, many of which are composed of atoms and their emergent properties, but also many of which are not. Contemporary examples of such immaterial phenomena include not only consciousness and other mental events but also such phenomena as justice, information, numbers, geometrical forms, the mathematical laws of nature, space, and time. Buddhism does not endorse materialism; neither does it embrace Cartesian dualism. It can rather be understood as a kind of empirical pluralism, recognizing that the natural world is far too rich to be categorized as being of only one or two types of substance. And unlike the Western scientific tradition, the Great Perfection, like the Middle Way view on which it is based, avoids the reification of any kind of substance—mental, material, or otherwise.

Upon investigating the nature of external and internal space by means of the practice of the Great Perfection, one discovers that these two spaces are also empty of any inherent nature. They are fabricated by conceptual imputations, and there is no objectively real boundary between them. This realization enables one to identify what is called the "mysterious space," which is the nonduality of external and internal space. A central aim of the Great Perfection is to maintain recognition of this nondual space of primordial consciousness not only while in meditation but also while actively engaging with the environment and other sentient beings. Dwelling in such a realization has been found to open up the reservoir of all-embracing, unconditional loving-kindness and compassion that is innate to the ultimate ground state of awareness. The distinction between wisdom and compassion has now vanished, and there is no bondage anywhere in sight.

All the previous practices of meditative quiescence, the four applications of mindfulness, the four immeasurables, and dream yoga are said to culminate in this one realization. Primordial consciousness is the alpha and omega of all such practice. Its gradual realization is the essence of the entire sequence of practices, and its perfect actualization is the final fruition. The immensely rich world of diverse natural phenomena, all arising as dependently related events, is seen as the play of this nonlocal awareness, which is fully present in each individual. Thus, according to this contemplative tradition, to know oneself is to know others. To know oneself is to know the whole of reality as an expression of the nondual wisdom and compassion of the clear light of awareness.

7

ŚAMATHA

THE CONTEMPLATIVE REFINEMENT OF ATTENTION

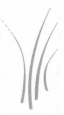

THE NATURE AND PURPOSE OF *ŚAMATHA*

Buddhist inquiry into the natural world proceeds from a radically different point of departure than Western science, and its methods differ correspondingly. As discussed previously, the pioneers of the scientific revolution, including Copernicus, Kepler, and Galileo, expressed an initial interest in the nature of the physical objects farthest removed from human subjectivity, such as the relative motions of the sun and earth, the surface of the moon, and the orbits of the planets. And a central principle of scientific naturalism is the complete objectification of the natural world, free of any contamination of subjectivity. This principle of objectivism demands that science deal with empirical facts testable by third-person means; such facts must, therefore, be public rather than private—accessible to more than one observer.

Another aspect of this principle is that scientific knowledge—paradigmatically, knowledge of astronomy and physics—must be epistemically objective, which is to say, observer-independent. A profound limitation of this ideal is that it cannot accommodate the study of subjective phenomena, which presumably accounts for the fact that the scientific study of the mind did not even begin until three hundred years after the launching of the scientific revolution. And it was roughly another hundred years before the nature of consciousness came to be accepted as a legitimate object of scientific inquiry. In short, the principle of objectivity excludes the subjective human mind and consciousness itself from the domain of natural science.

In stark contrast to this objective orientation, Buddhism begins with the premise that the mind is the primary source of human joy and misery and is central to understanding the natural world as a whole. In a well-known discourse attributed to the Buddha, he declares, "All phenomena are preceded by the mind. When the mind is comprehended, all phenomena are comprehended."[1] The mind and consciousness itself are therefore the primary subjects of introspective investigation within the Buddhist tradition. Moreover, just as unaided human vision was found to be an inadequate instrument for examining the moon, planets, and stars, Buddhists regard the undisciplined mind as an unreliable instrument for examining mental objects, mental processes, and the nature of consciousness.

Drawing from the experience of earlier Indian contemplatives, the Buddha refined techniques for stabilizing and refining the attention and used them in new ways, much as Galileo improved and utilized the telescope for observing the heavens. Over the 2,500 years since, Buddhist contemplatives have further developed and made use of those methods for training the mind, which they regard as the one instrument by which mental phenomena can be directly observed. As a result of their investigations, they have formulated elaborate, sophisticated theories of the origins and nature of consciousness and its active role in nature, but their inquiries have not produced anything akin to an empirical study or theory of the brain.

They did, however, develop rigorous techniques for examining and probing the mind firsthand. The initial problem was to train the attention so that it could be a more reliable, precise instrument of observation. Without such training, it is certainly possible to direct one's awareness inward, but the undisciplined mind has been found to succumb very swiftly to attentional excitation, or scattering; when it eventually calms down, it tends to drift into attentional laxity in which vividness is sacrificed. A mind that is alternately prone to excitation and laxity is a poor instrument for examining anything, and indeed, the Buddhist tradition deems it "dysfunctional."

Thus, the first task in the Buddhist investigation of the mind is to so refine the attention and balance the nervous system that the mind is made properly functional, free of the detrimental influences of excitation and laxity. Those two hindrances must be clearly identified in terms of one's own experience. Excitation, the first obvious interference in observing the mind, is defined as an agitated mental process that follows after attractive objects,[2] and it is a derivative of compulsive desire.[3] Laxity is a mental process that occurs when the attention becomes slack and the meditative object is not apprehended with vividness and forcefulness. It is said to be a derivative of delusion.

The genre of attentional training Buddhists have devised to counteract excitation and laxity is known as *śamatha*, the literal meaning of which is "quiescence." *Śamatha* is a serene attentional state in which the hindrances of excitation and laxity have been thoroughly calmed. The central goals of its cultivation are the development of attentional stability and acuity. In Buddhist psychology, the continuum of awareness is composed of successive moments, or "pulses," of cognition each lasting on the order of one millisecond.[4] Moreover, commonly in a continuum of perception, many moments consist of nonascertaining cognition, that is, moments in which objects *appear* to the inattentive awareness but are not *ascertained*, or consciously recognized so that they can be recalled later.[5]

In terms of this theory, I surmise that the degree of attentional stability increases in relation to the proportion of moments of ascertaining cognition of the intended object; that is, as stability increases, fewer and fewer moments are focused on any other object. This makes for a homogeneous continuum of perception. The degree of attentional vividness corresponds to the ratio of moments of ascertaining to nonascertaining cognition: the higher the frequency of the former, the greater the vividness. Thus, the achievement of *śamatha* entails an exceptionally high density of homogenous moments of ascertaining consciousness.

To return to the analogy of the telescope, the development of attentional stability may be likened to mounting a telescope on a firm platform; the development of attentional vividness is like highly polishing the lenses and bringing the telescope into clear focus. Recall the more traditional analogy, cited earlier, to illustrate the importance of attentional stability and vividness for the cultivation of contemplative insight: in trying to examine a hanging tapestry at night, if you light an oil lamp that is both radiant and unflickering, you can vividly observe the depicted images. But if the lamp is either dim or—even if it is bright—flickers due to wind, you cannot clearly see those forms.

THE USE OF A MENTAL IMAGE AS THE OBJECT IN *SAMATHA* PRACTICE

Among the wide variety of techniques devised for the cultivation of *śamatha*, one of the most commonly practiced among Tibetan Buddhist contemplatives entails focusing the attention upon a mental image. It may be of a visual object, such as a stick or a pebble, although Tibetan Buddhists tend to prefer mental images having great religious significance to them, such as an image of the Buddha.[6]

Regardless of the particular technique followed in the pursuit of *śamatha*, two mental faculties are said to be indispensable for the cultivation of attentional stability and vividness: mindfulness and introspection. The Pāli term translated here as "mindfulness" (*sati*) also has the connotation of "recollection," and it is the faculty of sustaining the attention upon a familiar object without being distracted. Thus, when using a mental image as the meditative object, mindfulness is applied steadily to it. Moreover, the image must be clearly ascertained, otherwise the full potency of attentional vividness cannot arise, subtle laxity is not dispelled, and concentration will remain flawed.

Mindfulness of a mental image is said to be a kind of mental perception. In the actual practice of *śamatha* it is common first to attend visually to an actual physical object, such as a pebble, and once one has grown thoroughly familiar with its appearance, to reconstruct a mental image of it and focus on that. In that phase of practice, mental perception apprehends the form of the pebble by the power of the visual perception of it. Thus, mental perception does not apprehend the pebble directly, but rather *recollects* it on the basis of the immediately preceding visual perception.

According to Buddhist psychology, the mental image of the pebble is not a mental faculty or process, for it does not cognize its own object, but neither is it material in the Buddhist sense of being composed of particles of matter. Rather, it is regarded as a form for mental consciousness,[7] of the same type as the forms that appear in the dream state. In this practice, mindfulness is focused on that mental image itself, not on the physical pebble of which the image is a likeness. In other words, it is the function of mindfulness to sustain the recollection of the image of the pebble, steadily observing it "internally" in a manner analogous to the visual observation of the pebble itself.

Mindfulness is the principal means of accomplishing *śamatha*, but it must be accompanied by the mental faculty of introspection. While mindfulness attends unwaveringly to the meditative object, introspection has the function of monitoring the meditative process. Thus, introspection is a type of metacognition that operates as the "quality control" in the development of *śamatha*, swiftly detecting the occurrence of either excitation or laxity. In the Buddhist tradition, introspection is defined as the repeated examination of the state of one's body and mind,[8] and it is regarded as a derivative of intelligence.[9]

The Buddhist assertion of the possibility of introspection as a form of metacognition raises the interesting problem of whether or not it is possible for the mind to observe itself. Buddhists generally assert that at any given moment, consciousness and its concomitant mental processes have the same intentional object, and at any given moment, only one consciousness can be produced in a single individual.[10] Moreover, a famous discourse attributed to the Buddha declares that the mind cannot observe itself, just as a sword cannot cut itself and a fingertip cannot touch itself; nor can the mind be seen in external sense objects or in the sense organs.[11]

I suspect the rationale behind that assertion is that even when one is aware of one's own subjective experience of an object, there is still a sense of separateness between the observer of that experience and the experience itself. The sense of duality remains. Within the context of ordinary, dualistic cognition, there can be no subjective awareness without an object, just as there can be no object without reference to a subject that cognizes or designates it. According to Tibetan Buddhist philosophy, subject and object are mutually interdependent. All phenomena experienced as subjects and objects arise within, and in dependence upon, the conceptual framework in which they are designated.

When one observes one's own subjective experience of an object, the observer seems to be distinct from that experience, and if one takes note of that observer, there remains a sense of duality between the noted observer and the one who notes that observer. This hypothesis of an observer perceiving a simultaneously existing observer perceiving a simultaneously existing observer leads to an infinite regression. Śāntideva avoided this problem by suggesting that instead of such metacognition occurring with respect to a simultaneously existing cognition, one is rather *recollecting* past moments of consciousness. In short, he hypothesized that it is possible to recollect a subjective experience that was not previously cognized as a distinct, isolated entity. In his view, when one remembers seeing a certain event, one recalls both the perceived event and oneself perceiving that event. The subject and object are recalled as an integrated, experienced event, in which the subject is retrospectively identified as such; but he denied that it is possible for a single cognition to take itself as its own object.[12]

THE STAGES OF DEVELOPMENT OF *ŚAMATHA*

Progress in the gradual training leading up to the achievement of *śamatha* is mapped out in terms of nine successive attentional states. The initial challenge is to develop a continuity of sustained, voluntary awareness, but in the first state, called "directed attention," the mind is strongly dominated by excitation. Indeed, because one is now consciously trying to sustain the attention unwaveringly on a single object instead of allowing it to roam freely, the mind seems more overwhelmed by compulsive ideation than usual. One brings the mental image to mind, but almost immediately it is lost and the attention is scattered.

This initial, limited capacity for sustained attention is borne out by modern experiments that have measured transient, focused attention on the basis of the performance of simple sensory tasks. Such research indicates that this transient, high level of focused attention lasts between one and three seconds.[13] Scientific investigation of attention during the late nineteenth century also suggested that voluntary attention cannot be sustained for more than a few seconds at a time. Such research led William James to conclude, "*No one can possibly attend continuously to an object that does not change.*"[14]

According to the Buddhist tradition, it is very difficult to attend continuously to an object that does not change, but the ability can be developed through sustained training. During the successive stages of *śamatha* practice, even the presence of mindfulness and introspection is no guarantee that progress will be made, for one may recognize the presence of laxity or excitation and still fail to take steps to counteract it. The remedy is the cultivation of the will, which is closely associated with intervention and effort. According to Buddhist psychology, the will is the mental process that intentionally engages the mind with various types of objects and activities. In this case, when either laxity or excitation occurs, the mind is stimulated by the will to intervene in order to eliminate them. The relationship of the mind to the will is likened to that of iron that moves under the influence of a magnet. The will to eliminate laxity and excitation is aroused by recognizing the disadvantages of succumbing to those hindrances and the advantages of overcoming them.[15] Thus, the initial two phases of this training are accomplished by learning about the nature of the practice and contemplating the benefits of pursuing it.

At the outset, one is encouraged to practice for many short sessions each day with as few distractions between sessions as possible. As a result of persevering in this practice, it is said that one ascends to the second state, called "continuous attention." During this phase, the mind is still subject to so much excitation that the attention is more often away from the object than on it, but at times one experiences brief periods of attentional continuity, for up to a minute or so. In other words, occasionally, for up to a minute, the attention does not completely disengage from the chosen mental image. But even during those periods of sustained attention, the mind is still prone to excitation, which manifests as peripheral "noise" or mental chitchat. Experientially, it seems as if the attention is still fixed on the mental image even while other thoughts and sensory impressions come to mind. According to Buddhist psychology, however, it seems more likely that the attention is disengaged from the mental image during those interludes, but they are so brief that there seems to be an unbroken continuity of attention to the main object. In any case, at this point only a gross level of attentional stability has been achieved, and that too is interspersed with periods of gross excitation, in which the meditative object is forgotten altogether.

With further training, one gradually reduces the number of sessions per day while increasing their duration. The emphasis is always on maintaining the highest quality of attention, rather than opting for mere quantity of time spent. The next state in this development is called "resurgent attention," at which point the attention is mostly on the meditative object, and its continuity needs only to be reinstated now and then when gross excitation occurs. Thus, there are more frequent periods of sustained attention, and they are of longer duration.

When one accomplishes the fourth state, called "close attention," the mind is stabilized to the point that one does not entirely disengage from the meditative object for the full duration of each session. The third and fourth states are achieved chiefly by the cultivation of mindfulness, and the principal emphasis up to that point is on the development of attentional stability, rather than vividness. In fact, Buddhist contemplatives have found that if one strives initially for enhanced vividness, that effort will actually undermine the development of stability. With the attainment of close attention, the power of mindfulness is well exhibited, gross attentional stability is achieved, and the mind is free of gross excitation.

Particularly at this point in the training, it is very easy to fall into complacency, a feeling of having already achieved the aim of sustained, voluntary attention. In reality, one is still very much subject to subtle excitation and to both gross and subtle laxity, and Tsongkhapa warns that if one fails to recognize these flaws, continued practice may actually impair one's intelligence. William James was also aware of pathological cases in which the mind was possessed by a fixed and ever monotonously recurring idea, and he mistakenly concluded that those were the only kind of cases in which the attention does become fixed on an unchanging object.[16] According to all the evidence available to him, voluntary attention is by necessity only a momentary affair.[17] Buddhist contemplatives maintain, on the contrary, that mental health can be retained and even enhanced as long as one cultivates a high degree of vividness in such sustained attention. The principal difference between such meditatively stabilized awareness and the kind of attention that occurs, for example, in obsessive-compulsive disorders is that the meditative awareness is voluntary and supple. It can be directed at will, instead of being obsessive or compulsive.

The fifth attentional state, called "tamed attention," and the sixth, called "pacified attention," are achieved with the force of introspection, with which one closely monitors the meditative process, watching for the occurrence of laxity and subtle excitation. In the stage of taming, gross laxity, in which vividness of the attention is missing, is dispelled; in the phase of pacification, subtle excitation is eliminated, so that even peripheral distractions disappear.

By that time, an increasing sense of joy and satisfaction arises while meditating, so the seventh and eighth attentional states of "fully pacified attention" and "single-pointed attention" are achieved by the force of enthusiasm. In the seventh state even subtle laxity, in which the full potency of attentional vividness is not attained, is eliminated; in single-pointed attention, the mind can dwell with utter stability and vividness on its chosen object for hours on end, without the occurrence of even subtle laxity or excitation. William James predicted that if the attention were concentrated on a mental image long enough, it would acquire before the mind's eye almost the brilliancy of a visually perceived object,[18] and this is exactly what Buddhist contemplatives report from their experience at this point of the training.

With the attainment of the ninth state, called "attentional balance," accomplished with the force of familiarization, only an initial impulse of will and effort is needed at the beginning of each meditation session; after that, uninterrupted, sustained attention occurs effortlessly. Moreover, the engagement of the will, effort, and intervention at this point is actually a hindrance. It is time to let the natural balance of the mind maintain itself without interference.

THE ATTAINMENT OF *SAMATHA*

Even at the state of attentional balance, *śamatha* has still not been fully achieved. Its attainment is marked first by a dramatic shift in the nervous system, characterized briefly by a strange but not unpleasant sense of heaviness and numbness on the top of the head. This is followed by an obvious increase in mental and then physical pliancy, entailing a cheerfulness and lightness of the mind and a buoyancy and lightness of the body. Consequently, experiences of physical bliss and then mental bliss arise, which are temporarily quite overwhelming. But that rapture soon fades, and with its disappearance, the attention is sustained firmly and calmly upon the meditative object, and *śamatha* is fully achieved. The above claims concerning a shift in the nervous system and its consequences have to do with firsthand, empirical, physiological experiences. It remains to be seen how, or whether, such a theory and the corresponding physiological changes can be detected objectively and understood in modern scientific terms.

With the achievement of *śamatha*, one disengages the attention from the previous meditative object, and the entire continuum of attention is focused single-pointedly, nonconceptually, and internally in the substrate consciousness, withdrawn fully from the physical senses. Thus, for the first time in this training, one does not attempt to recall a familiar object or mentally engage with it. One's consciousness is now left in an absence of appearances, an experience that is said to be subtle and difficult to realize. Only the aspects of the sheer awareness, luminosity, and joy of the mind remain, without the intrusion of any sensory objects. Any thoughts that arise do not persist, nor do they proliferate; rather, they vanish of their own accord, like bubbles emerging from water. One has no sense of one's own body, and it seems as if one's mind has become indivisible with space.

While remaining in this absence of appearances, even though it is still impossible for a single moment of consciousness to observe itself, one moment of consciousness may recall the experience of the immediately preceding moment, which, in turn, may recall its immediately preceding moment—each moment having no other appearances or objects arising to it. Thus, due to the homogeneity of this mental continuum, with each moment of consciousness recalling the previous one, the experiential effect is that of consciousness apprehending itself.

The defining characteristics of consciousness retrospectively perceived in that state are first a sense of *clarity*, or implicit luminosity capable of manifesting as all manner of appearances, and second the quality of *cognizance*, or the event of knowing. Upon attaining *śamatha*, by focusing the attention on the *sheer* clarity and the *sheer* cognizance of experience, one attends to the defining characteristics of consciousness alone, as opposed to the qualities of other *objects* of consciousness.

THE USE OF NONIDEATION AS THE OBJECT
IN *SAMATHA* PRACTICE

If one's chief aim in developing *samatha* is to ascertain the nature of consciousness, one might ask whether a more direct strategy—not engaging with a mental image or any other object—might be used. Many Buddhist contemplatives have in fact trained in an alternative technique of cultivating nonconceptual attention from the outset, without focusing on any other object such as a mental image. In this method the eyes are left open, gazing vacantly into the space ahead. According to Buddhist psychology, this space is a type of form that is apprehended by mental, not sensory, perception.[19] Mentally, one completely cuts off all thoughts of the past, future, and present. Bringing no thoughts to mind, one lets it remain like a cloudless sky, clear, empty, and evenly devoid of grasping onto any kind of object.

In this, as in all other techniques for the development of *samatha*, attentional stability and vividness are cultivated by means of mindfulness and introspection. The object of mindfulness is the mere absence of ideation, and with introspection one monitors whether the mind has come under the influence of excitation or laxity. Tsongkhapa especially emphasized that while following this method, one must *ascertain* the absence of ideation as the meditative object, rather than simply letting the mind go blank. His concern, I presume, was to ensure that the meditator does not drift into a nebulous trance but maintains an actively engaged intelligence throughout this training. In this way, one progresses through the nine attentional states explained previously. Eventually *samatha* is achieved, and—as in the previous method—it is characterized by joy, luminosity, and nonconceptuality.[20]

Buddhist contemplatives raise the question of whether this nonconceptual state of *samatha* actually transcends all conceptual structuring and modification and whether the mere suppression of ideation is sufficient for entering a totally nonconceptual state of awareness. The eminent Tibetan Buddhist contemplative Karma Chagmé (1612–1678) voiced the consensus within the Tibetan tradition when he asserted that although this state may easily be mistaken for conceptually unstructured awareness, it is not unmodified by ideation, for one still maintains the conceptual sense that attention is being sustained in the absence of conceptualization.[21]

Once *samatha* is achieved, the conceptually discursive mind becomes almost entirely quiescent. Only occasionally does an isolated thought or mental image fleetingly arise, only to fade back into the space of awareness, with no ripple effect. But even though one's awareness seems to be devoid of thoughts, there is still a subliminal sense of subject and object and other indications that this experience is subject to precognitive conceptual structuring. So the vacuum state of the mind of *śamatha* is relatively empty of conceptual content, but not absolutely so.

SETTLING THE MIND IN ITS NATURAL STATE

There is something contrived about the above state of nonconceptuality, for during the training that leads to it, the mind has been artificially withdrawn from appearances and ideation has been suppressed. The consciousness in which one perceives the characteristics of joy, luminosity, and nonconceptuality has been conceptually isolated from its normal processes and from the appearances with which it is normally engaged. The question may then be raised: Is it not possible to identify the natural characteristics of consciousness in the midst of the mind's activity, without suppressing ideation? After all, consciousness is obviously present and active while thoughts arise, so in principle there seems no reason it could not be identified.

It is for this purpose that the technique of "settling the mind in its natural state" has been devised and taught within the Indo-Tibetan Buddhist tradition.[22] Like all other techniques for developing *śamatha*, it entails freeing the mind from distraction, so that the attention is not compulsively carried away by either mental or sensory stimuli. However, this method is exceptional in that the attention is not fixed upon any object. One gazes steadily into the space ahead, but without visually focusing on anything. Mentally, one brings the attention into the domain of the mind, and whenever any type of mental event is observed—a thought, an image, a feeling, a desire, and so on—one simply takes note of it, without conceptually classifying it and without trying to suppress or sustain it. Letting the mind remain at ease, one watches all manner of mental events arise and pass of their own accord, without intervention of any kind. Settling awareness in the present, the attention is not allowed to stray in thoughts concerning the past or the future, or to latch onto any object in the present.

Normally when thoughts arise, one conceptually engages with the referents, or intentional objects, of those thoughts, but in this practice one perceptually attends to the thoughts themselves, without judging or evaluating them. The heart of the practice is allowing consciousness to remain in its "natural state," limpid and vivid, without becoming agitated in fluctuating emotions and habitual thought patterns.

While following this practice, one alternately seeks out the consciousness that is engaging in the meditation and then releases awareness. This is said to be an effective means of dispelling laxity. The First Panchen Lama, writing in the seventeenth century, described this as follows:[23]

> Whatever sort of thoughts arise, without suppressing them, recognize where they are moving and where they are moving to; and focus while observing the nature of those thoughts. By so doing, eventually their movement ceases and there is stillness.

The result of this practice is that flawless *samatha* arises, such that wherever the awareness is placed, it is unwaveringly present, unmoved by adventitious thoughts, and vividly clear, unsullied by laxity, lethargy, or dimness. In this way, too, the sheer clarity and cognizance of consciousness can be recognized.

THE ALLEGED TRAIT EFFECTS OF ACCOMPLISHING *SAMATHA*

In addition to various, valuable state effects of attaining *samatha*, mentioned earlier, a number of trait effects are also claimed by Buddhist contemplatives. Following such meditation, afflictive mental states such as aggression and craving are said to occur less frequently and to be of briefer duration than previously. Even when destructive mental processes arise, one does not readily succumb to them, and the mind remains calm and composed. Moreover, particularly as a result of settling the mind in its natural state, one experiences a nonconceptual sense that nothing can harm the mind, regardless of whether or not ideation has ceased. In between meditation sessions, when going about normal daily activities, one experiences a heightened sense of attentional vividness; it seems as if even sleep is suffused with exceptional concentration, and dream life takes on special significance. These claims are psychologically and physiologically significant, and they lend themselves to being tested scientifically so that we can understand more precisely what is meant by "attentional vividness" and the other purported shifts in consciousness while sleeping and dreaming.

Claims of extrasensory perception and paranormal abilities are quite common within the Buddhist tradition, in which no theoretical principles refute the possibility of such attainments and numerous methods are taught and practiced to acquire them. Recall the earlier cited statement of the Buddha: "All phenomena are preceded by the mind. When the mind is comprehended, all phenomena are comprehended." This is followed by an equally provocative assertion: "By bringing the mind under control, all things are brought under control."[24] Modern science has apparently assumed the opposite perspective: when the environment and the body, and specifically the brain, are brought under control, the mind is brought under control. In its pursuit of hedonic well-being, the modern West has sought techniques to control the environment and maintain fine physical health, and it has produced a stunning array of drugs to control the mind, enabling people to relax, to become mentally aroused and alert, to sleep, to relieve anxiety, to overcome depression, to counteract attentional disorders, to improve the memory, and to experience euphoria, bliss, and even alleged mystical states of consciousness.

While the modern Western approach is remarkably empowering for those who create, market, and distribute the above types of technology and drugs, it is profoundly disempowering for the individual. The Buddhist approach, with its emphasis on eudaimonic well-being, provides little incentive for the rigorous, sustained, extraspective investigation of physical processes and for the development of technology. Given the current, unprecedented encounter of the ancient Buddhist tradition and modern science, there is no reason we should be forced to choose one and exclude the other, although the question of which to emphasize more strongly is a matter of personal inclination.

The ultimate aim of the practice of *śamatha* is not simply to ascertain the primary characteristics of consciousness or to attain exceptional mental powers. Rather, it is to realize the nature of primordial consciousness. For exceptional individuals, the previously described method of settling the mind in its natural state may be sufficient for gaining such realization, but for most people, further training in the practice of the Great Perfection is required.[25]

PROLEGOMENA TO A FUTURE CONTEMPLATIVE SCIENCE

By the end of the nineteenth century, many physicists were utterly convinced that there were no more great discoveries to be made in their field—their understanding of the physical universe was complete in all important respects. One of the few lingering problems to be solved was known as the "ultraviolet catastrophe," which had to do with the incompatibility of entropy-energy formulas derived from classical thermodynamics. The solution to this problem came from Max Planck, who thereby laid the foundation for modern quantum theory, which shook the very foundations of physicists' views of the universe.[26]

While there is certainly no comparable sense that the cognitive sciences have formulated a comprehensive theory of the brain and mind—far to the contrary!—many experts in this field have concluded beyond a shadow of a doubt that consciousness is produced solely by the brain and that it has no causal efficacy apart from the brain. The fact that modern science has failed to identify the nature of consciousness, its necessary and sufficient causes, and its brain correlates in no way diminishes the certainty of those holding materialist views of the mind. When empirical knowledge of the nature and potentials of consciousness replaces these current metaphysical assumptions, I strongly suspect that the "problem of consciousness" will turn out to have a role in the history of science comparable to that of the ultraviolet catastrophe.

The most effective way to acquire such knowledge, I believe, is by a concerted, collaborative effort on the part of professional cognitive scientists and professional contemplatives, using their combined extraspective and introspective skills to tackle the hard problem of consciousness. This might involve, among other things, conducting longitudinal studies of the gradual development of *śamatha* by people devoting themselves to this training with the same dedication displayed by the scientists employed in the Genome Project. The successful completion of that effort to understand the genetic code is changing the face of the modern world. The collaborative scientific and contemplative study of *śamatha* may also help to restore a true spirit of empiricism to the study of consciousness and its relation to the world at large.

8

BEYOND IDOLATRY

THE RENAISSANCE OF A SPIRIT OF EMPIRICISM

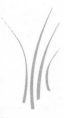 **THE PRIMARY OBSTACLE** to the spirit of empiricism in both religion and science is the deeply ingrained human tendency toward idolatry. My use of the term here is based on Francis Bacon's notion of an idol as a false absolute resulting from reification, in which we grasp for an absolute entity where there is none.

One sign of idolatry is a nonreciprocal coupling, or interaction, between two entities, in which the unaffected partner is identified as an idol. "Idols of the tribe," according to Bacon, are those common to a whole community, and historically they have cropped up in both religious and scientific contexts.[1] In contrast, the history of physics has time and again proven that the coupling among such phenomena as space, time, mass, and energy is reciprocal. This is not Newton's physical principle of action and reaction, but, as physicist David Finkelstein suggests, it might be its philosophical grandmother.[2] I shall now explore some of the primary idols of religion and of science and explore ways of overcoming them in order to restore a spirit of empiricism to both avenues of inquiry.

RELIGIOUS IDOLATRIES

The Idolization of the Self

According to the idolatry of "metaphysical individualism," the self is regarded as unchanging, unitary, and autonomous.[3] As a result of reifying such an absolutely separate, independent self, we similarly reify "the other," creating an absolute division between self and other and between subject and object in general. This idol of the self is invisible, assumed to exist as an absolutely subjective entity, outside the domain of experience, yet exerting its own autonomous free will on the body and the environment. This view has been formalized in certain philosophical systems, such as the philosophy of Descartes, who declared that the will is so free in its nature that it can never be constrained, yet the soul itself is unmoved.[4]

On the basis of this idolization of the self, we identify certain things, especially those over which we believe we exert control, as "mine," and reify this sense of ownership. In our pursuit of hedonic well-being, we may identify things such as wealth, power, fame, and cherished people as true sources of happiness and others as objective sources of misery. Instinctively wishing to experience pleasure and avoid pain, we respond with craving and attachment to these agreeable stimuli, and when anything obstructs our efforts to possess these objects or appears to inflict pain, we respond with anger and hatred as we regard them as true sources of our frustration and dissatisfaction.

Most cognitive scientists now generally refute the notion of an autonomous self, or homunculus, that exists independently from and controls the mind and brain, and many contemporary secular and religious philosophers have come to the same conclusion.[5] This does not necessarily imply that the self doesn't exist at all, but rather that it does not exist as an unchanging, unitary, autonomous entity.

Buddhism is perhaps the most prominent contemplative tradition to refute the existence of such an unchanging, unitary, independent self that autonomously controls the body and mind, but its refutation does not undermine the existence of selves altogether.[6] Conventionally, each of us does exist as a distinct person, living in interdependence with other sentient beings and the rest of the environment. And each of us is morally responsible for our actions, both individually and collectively.

Through the contemplative investigation of the true sources of happiness and suffering, Buddhists have found that none of these objects is intrinsically pleasurable. This is not to say that such objects do not contribute to happiness and suffering, but rather that they are not capable by themselves of producing those results. Having realized this, we may either fall into apathy and despair, feeling that the pursuit of happiness is futile, or begin to explore other avenues in our pursuit of genuine happiness, identifying its inner sources.

In the pursuit of hedonic pleasure, the more one person acquires in the way of such things as wealth, power, and fame, the less everyone else has, and this is an inevitable source of endless strife and conflict. In contrast, in the pursuit of eudaimonic well-being, one person's success in no way impairs or diminishes anyone else's well-being. On the contrary, it often serves as a source of inspiration and happiness for others. No wars have been fought over eudaimonic well-being, but countless wars have been fought over the objects of hedonic pleasure.

The Idolization of God

One of the clearest idolizations of God appears in Aristotle's *Metaphysics*, in which he described God as an "Unmoved Mover." Such a being, he argued, is the first principle because it causes all motion and is the basis of both heaven and nature.[7] God eternally does one thing—thinks—and because God thinks, God is alive. For this reason, life originates from God, for the actuality of life is thought. Moreover, Aristotle characterized God as a substance (*ousia*), but differentiated it from all other substances, insofar as it is "eternal, unmovable and separate from sensible things."[8]

Religious believers who have idolized this invisible God commonly view him as the one true source not only of eudaimonic well-being but also of hedonic pleasure. As the ultimate source, God is also the source of all misfortune, so he is frequently blamed for people's personal difficulties and for natural calamities. Such idolatry naturally promotes attachment to one's God as supreme and intolerance of those who do not believe in and revere him. This, in turn, leads to the perpetuation of violence between factions reifying and clinging to their own gods.

Late medieval Christian theology was heavily influenced by the Aristotelian view of God, but this view was gradually eroded by the advances of science. Especially since the nineteenth century, God has played little or no role in the scientific conception of the natural world. Einstein found any concept of a supreme deity fundamentally incompatible with science, and even declared that adherence to such an idol is the major source of conflict between religion and science.[9] But this position does not deny all notions of divinity, as Einstein himself declared his "firm belief, a belief bound up with a deep feeling, in a superior mind that reveals itself in the world of experience."[10]

Nevertheless, many contemporary philosophers reject all notions of God and an afterlife. John Searle writes, "In our deepest reflections we cannot take such opinions seriously. When we encounter people who claim to believe such things ... at bottom we remain convinced that either they have not heard the news or they are in the grip of faith."[11] Buddhism has always rejected the idea of a divine unmoved mover, and many contemplatives in other theistic and nontheistic traditions have also rejected the idea of God as an absolutely objective, independent being who exists apart from the world and controls it. Such a notion of God may be an extrapolation of the transcendental notion of the self, and both are idols that do not withstand empirical investigation or rational analysis.

SCIENTIFIC IDOLATRIES

The Idolization of the Brain

Many cognitive scientists believe that the brain influences the mind, but the subjectively experienced mind does not influence the brain. Fixing on the brain as an absolute in this mind-brain coupling puts it in the role of an idol. Neuroscientist Daniel M. Wegner adopts just such a view when he writes, "It seems to each of us that we have conscious will. It seems we have selves. It seems we have minds. It seems we are agents. It seems we cause what we do ... it is sobering and ultimately accurate to call all this an illusion."[12] In making this claim, he rejects not only the idol of the self but also the causal efficacy of the mind.

An implication of this stance is that the human mind and identity are reduced to the brain, which is regarded as the ultimate source of all happiness and sorrow, the sole place from which all pleasures and pains are generated. Therefore, to find greater happiness and freedom from suffering, the immediate path to success is through the manipulation of the brain. It is natural then to view psychopharmaceutical and psychotropic drugs as primary sources of happiness and relief from suffering. Medical doctors who adopt this view resist the notion that behavior and the mind influence the brain and body, and patients who accept it refuse to take personal responsibility for their health. This attitude results in a myriad of chronic diseases brought on by unhealthy diet and behavior, the symptoms of which are then "managed" with pharmaceutical drugs and other medical interventions. Another tragic consequence of this idolatry of the brain is the widespread disappearance of moral responsibility. If we were truly automatons programmed by our brains and genes, we would not accountable for our behavior, and the whole idea of punishment (and reward) should be abandoned.

If scientific evidence clearly indicates that the mind is a passive epiphe-nomenon of the brain, then we must accommodate that fact. But a careful examination of what is and is not known scientifically about the mind-brain problem shows that this issue is far from resolved. Benjamin Libet's well-known experiment[13] shows that subjects don't have the thought that they are consciously intending an action until some time after the brain activity underlying the action has begun. But this doesn't imply that those preced-ing brain activities weren't influenced by mental activity that preceded *them*. The same point holds true for Wegner's fundamental premise cited above.[14] Wegner has attended to brain mechanisms, looking to them alone for causal efficacy, and as James predicted, he does not count subjectively experienced choices as existing at all.

Wegner's claim to make any "ultimately accurate" statement about mind-body interactions seems especially overambitious in light of the lack of cur-rent scientific knowledge about how neural events influence mental events and vice versa. John Searle acknowledges that "We would ... need a much richer neurobiological theory of consciousness than anything we can now imagine to suppose that we could isolate necessary conditions of conscious-ness."[15] And he admits that he does not know why the necessary and suffi-cient causes of consciousness have not yet been identified.[16]

The consensus among cognitive scientists that the brain is solely respon-sible for the generation of all states of consciousness is remarkable in light of the facts that 1) they have no scientific means of detecting the presence of consciousness in anything; 2) they have no scientific definition of conscious-ness; 3) they have not identified the neural correlates of consciousness; and 4) they have not discovered the necessary and sufficient causes of conscious-ness. After more than a century of neurophysiological research, we are still in the dark regarding all these questions, so it is premature to presume, as Searle declares, that "Dualism in any form is today generally regarded as out of the question because it is assumed to be inconsistent with the scien-tific world view."[17] In light of the extent of scientific ignorance regarding the nature and origins of consciousness, when people claim that the problem of consciousness must necessarily be purely biological, to reflect Searle's com-ment back on his own position, such people either haven't heard the news or are in the grip of faith. As Mark Twain cautioned, "It ain't what you don't know that gets you in trouble. It's what you know for sure that just ain't so."

Many cognitive scientists assume that if subjective mental experience were anything other than brain function, it could not possibly influence the brain or any other physical entity. This, they believe, is the unavoidable implication of the closure principle, which states that there are no nonphysical influences in the physical world. As discussed previously, this principle is based on nineteenth-century classical physics, which heralded the conservation of energy as the key for understanding nature as a whole. However, the closure principle must be reconsidered within the context of quantum mechanics, which does not support it as an absolute, invariable law of nature. Indeed, the more physics progresses, the more it appears to undermine previously held, absolute laws of conservation.[18] According to quantum theory, the "energy-time uncertainty principle" does allow for violations of energy conservation, so it is possible in principle for nonphysical processes to influence matter. As physicist Paul C. W. Davies writes, "One expression of the uncertainty principle is that physical quantities are subject to spontaneous, unpredictable fluctuations. Thus energy may surge out of nowhere; the shorter the interval the bigger the energy excursion."[19] Whether such violations of energy conservation are relevant to brain activity is an open question that is presently being investigated by physicists and biologists. Another relevant, unresolved issue is the location of information that is stored in the brain. If it turns out that information is stored at the atomic level, this could imply that quantum effects are present in the brain. This requires further research.

The notion that the mind is passive, whatever its ontological status may be, has been thoroughly discredited by science. One of the clearest indications of this is the euphemism of the so-called "placebo effect." I call this a euphemism because a placebo refers to a substance or treatment with no known effect on the condition being studied. Therefore, the effects that are observed, evidently caused by such mental processes as expectation, desire, hope, belief, and trust, are nominally attributed to something that is specifically designed *not* to affect the condition being studied. The "nocebo effect" refers to the opposite: people expect they will experience something painful or afflictive, and that's just what they get. In this case, their thoughts, emotions, and beliefs cause physical effects, but how these mind-body causal interactions occur is far from clear.

The size of the placebo effect varies from study to study and depends on the condition under investigation, but 35 percent is a frequently cited figure, while in some cases it is far higher. In 1998, Irving Kirsch, who has done provocative work in this area, stirred up a lot of controversy with his paper "Listening to Prozac But Hearing Placebo: A Meta-Analysis of Antidepressant Medication."[20] More recent research reveals not only that 50 to 75 percent of the efficacy of antidepressant medication is due to the placebo effect but also that "effective" placebo treatment induces changes in brain function that are distinct from those associated with antidepressant medication.[21] An even more mysterious proposition that is almost certainly true is that sometimes placebos catalyze novel kinds of somatic experiences, rather than simply replications of previous symptoms. In some documented cases, mental effects (let's finally call them what they are) actually override the effects of physiologically active drugs.

In cases where the mind catalyzes unprecedented effects in the body, the nature of the mind-body interaction is especially mysterious. How is it that an individual with no knowledge of brain mechanisms or physiology can mentally cause changes in the body corresponding to an uninformed belief or expectation? Neuroscientists commonly believe that information is stored in higher orders of organization of neuronal networks. Maybe so. But how, exactly? In the case of information stored in a computer, Searle points out, "The information in the computer is in the eye of the beholder, it is not intrinsic to the computational system.... The electrical state transitions of a computer are symbol manipulations only relative to the attachment of a symbolic interpretation by some designer, programmer or user."[22] If the brain is accurately portrayed as a biological computer, where is the outside "eye of the beholder," and what is the nature of the designer, programmer, or user? An alternative hypothesis is that information is actually stored in the mind, which acts as a substrate for certain neural events, rather than the other way around. As we shall see in the next section, the status of information in relation to the material world is a question physicists are grappling with today, sometimes proposing startling hypotheses.

Wherever information is stored, the undisputed prevalence of placebo effects incontrovertibly refutes the hypothesis that in the relationship between the mind and brain, the mind is a passive partner. Instances of the placebo effect are far from unique in this regard. Other studies show that mental training modifies neural networks, coordinates regional brain oscillations, and modifies neurosecretory functions. The recent work of Antoine Lutz, Richard Davidson, and their colleagues has received a good deal of public attention.[23] All such research shows that the idol of the brain has been toppled by empirical evidence. But there is one more idol to throw down, and this one is embedded in the foundations of scientific materialism.

The Idolization of Nature

Most members of the National Academy of Science now refute the idol of a God who exists apart from and controls the universe,[24] but just as Descartes's idol of the soul has been replaced by the idol of the brain, so has the idol of God been replaced by the idol of Nature. The current idolatry of Nature finds its historical precedent in Descartes's declaration that "there exists nothing in the whole of nature which cannot be explained in terms of purely corporeal causes, totally devoid of mind and thought."[25] According to this view, the absolutely objective world of matter, transcending the subjective realm of sensory appearances and invisible to human perception, is causally closed: it generates all subjective appearances of the objective world but is uninfluenced by them. Much as Aristotle attributed thought and life to the Unmoved Mover, so do advocates of scientific materialism claim that life, intelligence, and consciousness all derive from the objective, physical world, which has been equated with Nature. In this way, Nature, comprised of space-time and mass-energy, has been made an idol, in a nonreciprocal coupling between two entities: objective physical phenomena and subjective mental phenomena. The material world is the unaffected partner, so it has been turned into an idol.

Some of the practical repercussions of such idolatry are the reification of the world of matter as the sole reality, together with the marginalization of all kinds of causal influences that cannot be identified within the world of physical mechanisms. This may account for the misnomer of the "placebo effect" in a worldview where only physical processes are supposed to exert any kind of influence. The idol of matter, like the divine idol that preceded it, is seen by its followers as the true source of all happiness and sorrow, all good fortune and adversity. Such a belief implies that one should seek happiness solely through the manipulation of the physical world, including inanimate objects and animate beings. Insatiable consumerism is a natural consequence of this idolatry, and with the limitless pursuit of limited material resources, the degradation of the environment and conflict—from interpersonal strife to international warfare—inevitably follow. The very notions of eudaimonic well-being and virtue are alien to this worldview.

Philosophically, this view of matter may be traced as far back as Democritus, who declared that in the objective world only atoms moving in space exist. A competing view was proposed by the Pythagoreans, who maintained that all things are numbers, which they identified with geometrical forms. Plato built on this notion by proposing that the world of appearances emerges from an underlying realm of pure ideas. Although physics throughout the nineteenth century appeared to corroborate the view of Democritus, with the advent of the twentieth-century revolution in physics, Werner Heisenberg concluded, "*With regard to this question, modern physics takes a definite stand against the materialism of Democritus and for Plato and the Pythagoreans.*"[26]

The scientific idolatry of Nature received major impetus from Hermann von Helmholtz's 1847 formulation of the principle of the conservation of energy and his assertion that it was the key to the complete comprehensibility of nature.[27] This hypothesis appeared to be strongly bolstered by Einstein's famous 1905 equation $E = mc^2$, but the issue seems more uncertain when we recall that according to Richard Feynman, the conservation of energy is a mathematical principle, not a description of a mechanism or anything concrete, and no one really knows what energy *is*.[28]

If Nature does not fundamentally consist of discrete units of matter, what is it made of? Physicist John Archibald Wheeler has proposed that reality exists not because of physical particles but rather because of the act of observing the universe. "Information may not be just what we *learn* about the world," he says. "It may be what *makes* the world."[29] In classical physics, when an ideal experimenter determines the state of a system, the state influences the experimenter, who learns something, but the experimenter does not influence the state, which is fixed. The state is the absolute. But, as Wheeler asserts, in quantum mechanics, "No elementary phenomenon is a phenomenon until it is a recorded phenomenon."[30] For this reason, quantum mechanics has been characterized as a "nonobjective physics," suggesting that it is founded not on objects but on interactions.[31]

With the advances of modern physics, the idol of Nature appears to be crumbling at its foundations. It is uncertain whether the world of subjective experience has physical attributes (is there any reason to believe that dreamscapes consist of configurations of mass-energy?), and it is also not clear that the objective world, independent of all systems of measurement, conforms to the notion of "physical." Even if it does, to whose notion of physical and to whose theory of matter does it conform? In terms of classical physics, a material body may be defined as a fraction of space endowed with constitutive properties such as impenetrability and mass. More conservatively, it may be said that a material entity is something that is permanently located in space, causally connected to changes in its spatial environment, and endowed with mass. But as philosopher Michel Bitbol argues, these three criteria are threatened by quantum mechanics, which challenges the primitive concept of matter as a collection of inherently massive and spatially defined particulate bodies.[32] Michael Lockwood posits a subtler definition of matter: "those things are material that occupy or take place in space, and whose existence is ultimately constituted by the properties and relations, actions and interactions of particles and fields, or whatever basic entities physics treats of."[33] In light of this sophisticated definition, it appears that mental phenomena, such as dreams, have no place in the material world unless they are found to be equivalent to neural events. But such an equivalence has never been demonstrated.

There are two worlds that are invisible to the third-person methodology of scientific inquiry: the absolutely objective world and the absolutely subjective world. What's left over is the world in between: the world of experience, which is directly ascertainable with our six senses, including our five physical senses (enhanced and extended with the instruments of technology) and mental perception.[34] Strictly speaking, when we observe subjective phenomena (such as thoughts, emotions, and dreamscapes) and objective phenomena (such as electrons, apples, and galaxies), all that directly appears to our senses are impressions generated in part by our brains. Those impressions do not consist of regions of space endowed with constitutive properties such as impenetrability and mass, nor are they constituted by the properties and relations, actions, and interactions of particles and fields. So none of the immediate contents of our experience conforms to any of the definitions of matter cited above. Matter, then, seems to be a conceptual construct that is superimposed upon the world of experience, which is immaterial.

This reframes the entire question of the nature of the universe, which many scientists define as physical.[35] The laws of nature, which were first formulated by Newton, are as exact and true as anything known in physics, yet they vanish into nothingness when examined very closely, while quantum-mechanical matter is found to consist of waves of nothing.[36] In this regard, it may be somewhat daunting to follow the implications of Robert Laughlin's assertion that "In physics, correct perceptions differ from mistaken ones in that they get clearer when the experimental accuracy is improved."[37]

While neurobiologists insist that the mind be explained in terms of biology and experimental physicists insist that biology be explained in terms of physics, mathematical physicists insist that physics be explained in terms of mathematics. But the realm of mathematics, like the realm of ideas in general, seems to be inseparable from the mind. So this succession brings us full circle! This suggests that there is a hierarchy in the sciences that challenges the widespread reductionist paradigm:[38]

- Mathematical theories alone do not define, predict, or explain the emergence of a physical universe.
- Physical theories alone do not define, predict, or explain the emergence of living organisms in the universe.

- Biological theories alone do not define, predict, or explain the emergence of consciousness in living organisms.

According to David Finkelstein, in Galilean physics, there is no space separate from time, so in the coupling of space and time, in which there is absolute time but no absolute space, time is an idol.[39] Likewise, in Newtonian physics and special relativity, space-time acts on matter but matter exerts no influence on space-time, so space-time becomes the idol. In the general theory of relativity, space-time and matter are found to be interdependent, and neither is any more fundamental than the other. So space-time can exist and change in the absence of anything previously called matter. Following this same development in the history of science, it may be necessary to challenge the common assumption that consciousness plays a secondary, subservient role in nature as a epiphenomenal, emergent property of matter. It may well be that consciousness, like space-time, has its own intrinsic degrees of freedom, and that neglecting them will lead to a description of the universe that is fundamentally incomplete. In short, our consciousness of the universe may be as real as the space-time and mass-energy of which we are conscious.[40]

The real world that we *know* exists is experienced within intersubjective fields of consciousness, in which mental phenomena are just as real as physical phenomena. And neither class of phenomena is simply a derivative of the other: neither is an idol. We now can finally extricate ourselves from the absolute dualism of Descartes, in which a reified objective world is absolutely separated from a reified subjective world, and return to the world of experience, in which those demarcations are recognized as human, conceptual constructs. Materialists, for all their adamant rejection of Cartesian dualism, continue to accept half of Descartes's bifurcated universe—the objective, material, mechanical half—and then try to reduce the other half—the subjective, immaterial, qualitative half—into the portion they have idolized. But an alternative is to go a step further by rejecting both halves of this reified, dualistic view of reality, and accept instead a participatory world of subject-object interdependence and interaction.

The Idolization of Theories

More fundamental than the religious idolization of the self and God and the scientific idolization of the brain and Nature is the idolization of theories to which all human communities are prone. David Finkelstein clarifies how this occurs: "One may think of any whole theory as a view, as etymology suggests. A view is a view from a position, which is then an idol of that theory. It seems that the process of making a theory inevitably introduces idols that only a later theory can break, and so the theory process can never be completed."[41] A position, or stance, is primarily a way of behaving, involving an interpretative orientation and a commitment to act and understand events in accordance with it. So it implies a kind of "epistemic policy" that is adopted in defining what counts as facts.[42]

In any encounter between scientific and contemplative stances, we repeatedly confront the intriguing question: What constitutes evidence, or empirical facts? As Robert Laughlin points out, "Physics maintains a time-honored tradition of making no distinction between unobservable things and nonexistent ones."[43] But are only objective observations to be considered as legitimate? While science relies overwhelmingly on third-person, objective observations, if it completely rejected first-person experience as evidence, there would be no empirical grounds for asserting the existence of mental phenomena, in which case the mind would have no place in nature. Until now, cognitive scientists have counted as evidence primarily the experiences of normal and subnormal people. Contemplatives, on the other hand, have an epistemic policy of counting the exceptional experiences of advanced meditators as the most important kind of evidence. The Dalai Lama has long taken the position that he is willing to reject any Buddhist assertion, such as belief in reincarnation, that is invalidated by scientific evidence.[44] But it is a rare scientist who is willing to reject any scientific assertion, such as a materialist interpretation of consciousness, if it is invalidated by contemplative evidence.

One of the primary consequences of the idolization of theories is the conflation of reality with one's perspective on reality, while remaining oblivious of the limitations of the position on which that perspective is based. This commonly results in disdain and intolerance toward anyone who holds views incompatible with one's beliefs, which all too frequently erupts in ideological warfare waged from pulpits, in schools, and on battlefields, as well as terrorist and military assaults on whole societies. For millennia, this has been a worldwide cause of religious wars, and in the more recent past, scientific materialists, often waving the banner of communism, have committed countless atrocities, sometimes amounting to genocide, against people who maintained their traditional religious beliefs despite the most brutal attempts to convert them to the ideology of materialism.

As Thomas Kuhn argued decades ago, human worldviews, scientific and otherwise, are always influenced by the societal context of the people developing and advocating those views.[45] And Robert Laughlin comments more recently, "Scientific theories always have a subjective component that is as much a creation of the times as a codification of objective reality."[46] But as long as we remain surrounded by people who adopt the same view from the same stance, it is difficult to identify our invisible, unsubstantiated assumptions and idols. A practical way to discover these hidden absolutes lurking within our belief systems is to engage with people whose ways of exploring reality are radically different. Regardless of how diverse their views may be, if common rules of logic and standards of empirical rigor can be found, meaningful collaboration may occur. In this regard, the Dalai Lama proposes a rational and empirical ideal that may be adopted by scientists and contemplatives alike: "A general basic stance of Buddhism is that it is inappropriate to hold a view that is logically inconsistent. This is taboo. But even more taboo than holding a view that is logically inconsistent is holding a view that goes against direct experience."[47]

Scientists and contemplatives of various traditions set out on their quest for truth using different sets of assumptions and methods of inquiry. Given the diversity of their ideological and methodological stances, any convergence of their views would be noteworthy, for it would be strong evidence that their conclusions transcend the limitations of their sociological contexts. So let us now examine whether any such deep convergence may have happened between the frameworks of science and two Buddhist and Christian traditions of contemplative inquiry.

CONVERGENCE

As noted repeatedly throughout this book, the first revolution in the physical sciences was brought about by such figures as Copernicus, Kepler, Descartes, Galileo, and Newton, who were all seeking a "God's-eye perspective" on the objective world as it exists independently of human consciousness. All these men were devout Christians well versed in theology, and Newton spent the last twenty-five years of his life writing more on theology than he did on science. In fact, he commented that he wrote his classic work *Mathematical Principles of Natural Philosophy* with an eye for principles that might cause people to believe in God.[48] The aspiration of these scientific pioneers was to come to know the mind of the creator by understanding his creation, and they drew an absolute demarcation between the objective world known by God and the subjective world perceived and conceived by humans. This theological stance gave rise to the Cartesian dualism of an absolutely objective world that is "represented" by subjective human percepts and concepts.

One fundamental assumption they held was that, although scientists are human subjects, with the faculty of reason they could infer the existence of objects and their qualities in the objective world on the basis of appearances to their senses, often enhanced by technological instruments of observation. There is an epistemological flaw, though, in this kind of reasoning. As Kant pointed out, we don't know that our sensory experiences resemble the external world if we have no means of knowing the external world as it exists independently from our experiences.

Quantum physicists have already run into the inconceivability of the nature of quantum entities existing independently of measurement, but the same problem crops up when trying to conceive of the true vacuum, which is defined as whatever remains once we have removed from some well-defined space everything that *the laws of nature* permit us to take away. The true vacuum, defined in this way, is distinguished from the false vacuum, which is whatever remains once we have removed from some well-defined space everything that the *current state of technology* permits us to take away. The problem with conceiving of the true vacuum is that scientists have not yet discovered all the laws of nature. In the perfect symmetry of the true vacuum, which is devoid of any internal structure, quarks, electrons, gravity, and electricity are undifferentiated. In the words of science writer K. C. Cole, "The closest we can probably come to imagining perfect symmetry is a smooth, timeless, featureless empty space—the proverbial blank slate, the utter silence. It can't be perceived because nothing can change. Everything would be one and the same; everything would be the same, as far as we could tell, as nothing."[49]

Both the false and the true vacuums in physics are thought to be devoid of consciousness, but this was a foregone conclusion since physicists have always sought to understand the natural world as it exists independently of human consciousness. Scientists have no means of objectively detecting consciousness, human or divine, so they have no way of knowing whether any kind of consciousness existed before the evolution of life, either on our planet or elsewhere. So the belief that consciousness can only have existed after the emergence of life on our planet is simply an assumption, and one that is now beginning to be questioned by a growing group of physicists.[50]

In the world of contemporary physics, bodies of mass in a vacuum are regarded metaphorically as "frozen energy," and they cause a curvature of space, such that the distance between two points in space also fluctuates. Configurations of mass and energy can be considered, in this sense, excitations of the vacuum, much as surface waves in a pond are excitations of the pond's water. While the vacuum itself is shapeless, it may assume specific shapes, and in doing so it becomes a physical reality, a "real world." So the true vacuum may have played a central role in the formation of the universe, in which at the time of the Big Bang the freezing of the true, or "melted," vacuum gave rise to the universe as we presently know it.[51]

As mentioned previously, the absolute space of phenomena is said to play a similar cosmogonic role in the Great Perfection tradition, which also uses the metaphor of a primordial ground "freezing" into the appearance of ordinary reality. The nineteenth-century classic *The Vajra Essence* declares,[52]

This ground is present in the mind-streams of all sentient beings, but it is tightly constricted by dualistic grasping; and it is regarded as external, firm, and solid. This is like water in its natural, fluid state freezing in a cold wind. It is due to dualistic grasping onto subjects and objects that the ground, which is naturally free, becomes frozen into the appearances of things.

In the practice of the Great Perfection, one comes to realize how all phenomena spontaneously emerge as empty, intangible, nonobjective configurations of space, and this all-pervasive domain is perceived as not separated from primordial consciousness. *The Vajra Essence* concludes, "Primordial consciousness is self-originating, naturally clear, free of outer and inner obscuration; it is the all-pervasive, radiant, clear infinity of space, free of contamination."[53]

The description of the true vacuum in modern physics makes it look like another version of an Unmoved Mover, an absolute dimension of reality that influences the phenomenal world but is uninfluenced by it. In other words, one more idol. According to the view of the Great Perfection, however, the absolute space of phenomena transcends all human conceptual categories, including those of permanence and impermanence and even existence and nonexistence. Words are useful only insofar as they lead one to the direct realization of ultimate reality. While absolute space is conventionally viewed as being existent, it cannot exist independently from relative space, and relative space cannot exist without absolute space. Likewise, the unity of primordial consciousness and the absolute space of phenomena does not exist independently of the phenomenal world but rather permeates it as the "one taste" of all phenomena.

In all kinds of interactions between two phenomena or classes of phenomena, idols creep in as a result of failing to attend to and comprehend one of the partners in those interactions. In scientific and contemplative inquiry, one unveils the idol of the self by closely examining one's own and others' bodies and minds, together with their interactions with the environment. To unmask the idol of God, one carefully observes the orderly patterns of dependently related events within the natural world and how they pertain to one's understanding (if any) of the divine. To expose the idol of the brain, one investigates the causal efficacy of subjectively experienced mental processes; and to reveal the idol of Nature, one scrutinizes the causal interactions of subjective experience with objective reality.

Likewise, to lay bare the idols of theories, one investigates the influences on the position, or stance, from which those theories are created and adopted. In the cases of science and religion, for instance, this means carefully studying the nonscientific and nonreligious influences on those worldviews, including all manner of subjective individual and cultural participation. For the moment, what we attend to is reality, and that reality is prone to become an idol when we fail to attend to the influences on it.

In short, Buddhism throws down the idols of the self, God, the brain, and Nature, replacing them with an all-pervasive view of dependent origination. Let us now apply the view of the Great Perfection to the scientific concepts of space-time, mass-energy, and body-mind. The absolute space of phenomena is pervaded not only by primordial consciousness but also by the infinite, vital energy of that consciousness (*jñāna-prāṇa*),[54] and it is also of the same nature as "the fourth time," a dimension of time that transcends the past, present, and future.[55] So relative space-time, mass-energy, and body-mind emerge from the ultimate symmetry of the absolute space of phenomena, the fourth time, primordial consciousness, and the energy of primordial consciousness, all of which are coextensive and of the same nature. These two sets of ultimate and relative phenomena have no inherent identities of their own apart from the conceptual frameworks in which they are conceived or apart from each other. In the mindful awareness of a world of dependent origination, there is no place for idols of any kind.

Many of the initial assumptions of Christian theology are as different from Buddhism as those of Buddhism are different from science. We have already noted some provocative similarities between scientific and Buddhist views of empty space, so let us now review some of the comparable conclusions drawn by Neoplatonic Christian contemplatives, beginning in the ninth century with John Scotus Eriugena. According to this view, *nihil*, or nothingness, transcends all phenomena, which all emerge from this Divine Essence.[56] Through contemplation, this transcendent good is seen to ineffably descend into the world of nature and is present in all things, with this ultimate reality proceeding by the power of thought from nothing to something. In this way, all phenomena are expressions of a theophany, consisting of appearances of the divine.

Nicholas of Cusa similarly explained the path of seeking God within oneself, resulting in the removal of all limits.[57] He described the ascent of the soul to God in this way:[58]

> I experience how necessary it is for me to enter into the cloud and to admit the coincidence of opposites, above all capacity of reason, and to seek there the truth where impossibility confronts me. And above reason, above even every highest intellectual ascent when I will have attained to that which is unknown to every intellect and which every intellect judges to be the most removed from truth, there are you, my God, who are absolute necessity.

Similar descriptions of ultimate reality are expressed in the contemplative writings of Judaism, Islam, Hinduism, and Taoism, which is remarkable in light of the many significant differences in the original doctrines of each of these world religions. These brief allusions to apparent similarities among modern physics, Buddhism, and Christianity are far from conclusive, but they do suggest a possible deep convergence toward a truth that transcends our ordinary experience of the world.[59] These topics call for thorough, comparative analysis, and if it turns out that there are truths on which science and the great contemplative traditions of the world come together, those may be the most important truths that can be known by humanity.

CONCLUSION

If the above theories of the vacuum of modern physics, the absolute space of phenomena of Buddhism, and the nothingness of Christianity do in fact converge, we may be tempted to view their synthesis as another attempt at a grand unified theory, which would present us with one more idol. All objects of knowledge—both perceptual and conceptual—tend to become idols due to the deeply ingrained tendency to reify everything we experience. To see through the idols, we must recognize that all objects of perception arise in interdependence with the perception of them, and all conceived objects, including theoretical entities such as fields and elementary particles, arise in interdependence with the conceptual framework in which they are conceived. The very categories of mind and matter, space and time, and mass and energy are human, conceptual constructs superimposed on the world of experience, and they have no existence apart from the conceptual frameworks in which they are conceived.

When it comes to trying to determine the validity of our experiences and ideas, it is important to recognize the impossibility of discovering whether any isolated moment of cognition is valid without reference to another moment of cognition. In other words, no single moment of awareness can stand alone as an absolutely valid cognition. By implication, it may be that no single mode of investigation—scientific or otherwise—can stand alone as the one absolutely valid means of knowledge. This implies that we must engage in a bootstrapping process in both scientific and contemplative inquiry, in which a discovery must be subjected to peer review and replication in order to be validated.

Another way to evaluate knowledge is to apply the criterion of pragmatism, for the value of our knowledge also hinges on the question: What is it good for?[60] This is a compelling rationale for bringing together very different disciplines, each having different working assumptions, goals, and methodologies. Cross-referencing them may more easily reveal their hidden assumptions, and perhaps also deep truths. A starting point for such comparative analysis may be to acknowledge the value of science for knowing the objective world and for enhancing hedonic well-being, while recognizing the value of the world's contemplative traditions for revealing the nature of the world of experience and enhancing eudaimonic well-being. The worlds explored by scientists and contemplatives are mutually interdependent, as are hedonic and eudaimonic well-being.

Over the past four hundred years, the physical sciences have undergone two major revolutions, the first in the seventeenth century and the second in the twentieth century. This second revolution is not yet complete, for no one has yet formulated a compelling unification of quantum mechanics and general relativity. A missing component that may be crucial for devising such a unified theory is an understanding of the role of the observer, which has thus far eluded physicists.[61] The biological sciences have undergone one major revolution, begun by Darwin in the mid-nineteenth century and culminating in the Genome Project in the late twentieth century. All those revolutions were based on the rigorous and precise observation of physical and biological phenomena.

The cognitive sciences have yet to undergo a single revolution. The direction of psychology proposed by William James, with its empirical emphasis on introspection, was stifled by the domination of scientific materialism over the past century. A major reason for this delay, which resulted from the failure to follow James's lead, is that cognitive scientists have yet to devise any rigorous and precise introspective methods for observing mental phenomena. Consequently, the materialistic assumptions about the nature and origins of consciousness that constituted the "popular view" among nonphilosophers since the time of Socrates remain unchallenged by modern science. Because of a dogmatic allegiance to the principles of scientific materialism, empirical methods for studying the mind have been confined mostly to verbal interrogation and the examination of the neural and behavioral correlates of mental phenomena. The first-person observation of these states of consciousness has been left to amateurs with no professional training in observing, experimenting with, or reporting on mental processes.

The revolutions in the physical and life sciences occurred only because scientists were willing to overthrow unsubstantiated beliefs when they conflicted with empirical discoveries, many of which occurred because of the development of increasingly sophisticated means of observation. One of the most prominent unsubstantiated beliefs in the current scientific study of the mind is that all states of consciousness are functions of the brain and have no existence apart from it. To determine whether this is true, we would need to know the full spectrum of all states of consciousness, like knowing the full spectrum of electromagnetic radiation before making broad generalizations about the nature of light. But, as mentioned before, the cognitive sciences have thus far confined their investigations almost entirely to the medium and low "bandwidth" of human consciousness. Within that range, it appears very likely that all states of consciousness are dependent on the brain. But Buddhist contemplatives have been principally interested in developing "high-energy" states of consciousness, in which *samādhi*, the primary "technology" of contemplative inquiry, plays a crucial role. In contemplative as well as scientific inquiry, truth and measurement technology are inextricably linked.[62] Since the possibility of the higher-frequency range of consciousness has hardly been considered by cognitive scientists, such states have never been factored into the scientific account of the mind.

When researchers do turn their attention to such highly developed modes of awareness, investigating them from both third-person and first-person perspectives in collaboration with highly advanced contemplatives, the scientific understanding of the mind may shift from classical mind-body relationships to relativistic ones. Buddhist contemplatives have long maintained that the participatory nature of the mind is revealed most clearly when the mind is empowered by the unified cultivation of meditative quiescence (*śamatha*) and contemplative insight (*vipaśyanā*). This is a hypothesis that can be tested experientially, setting aside all dogmas and commitments to unsubstantiated beliefs, scientific or religious. As Robert B. Laughlin comments, "Seeing through ideologies and debunking them is what real science is all about. Mental life in general, I think."[63] This is certainly a central aim of both contemplative and scientific inquiry at their best, and it requires unflinching allegiance to the spirit of empiricism. But such a renaissance in the cognitive sciences will not come easily. As philosopher Bas van Fraassen remarks, "Being or becoming an empiricist will then be similar or analogous to conversion to a cause, a religion, an ideology."[64]

Descartes bequeathed to humanity an egocentric view of the mind, and modern cognitive scientists are committed to a neurocentric view. The rejection of the idols of the mind and the brain may result in a shift of perspective on the mind-body problem to one of dependent origination, with both partners in the coupling participating in a relationship of mutual interdependence. Aristotle left a theocentric view of the world, and modern physicists are committed to a physiocentric view. The rejection of the idols of God and Nature may give way to a reassessment of the whole of reality as being of dependent origination, in which all subjective and objective phenomena are interdependently related. Physicist Nick Herbert comments that the source of all quantum paradoxes seems to lie in the fact that human perceptions create a world of unique actualities—our experience is inevitably "classical"—while quantum reality is simply not that way at all. And he asks, "Since physics assures us that our lives are embedded in a thoroughly quantum world, is it so obvious that our experience must remain forever classical?"[65] To this question, contemplatives throughout history have responded with a resounding "No!"

Science has provided multiple conceptual revolutions in our way of viewing reality, but these have had little impact on the cultivation of genuine happiness or virtue. The contemplative traditions of the world have provided multiple experiential revolutions in ways of viewing reality, which have directly altered the hearts, minds, and lives of those who have acquired such contemplative insights and indirectly influenced their host societies. But contemplative inquiry has left humanity in the dark about many truths pertaining to the physical world, and has yielded no advances in technology. In short, these two approaches to understanding appear to be fundamentally complementary, rather than incompatible.

In our modern world, the pursuits of happiness, truth, and virtue have been widely regarded as unrelated and even opposed. With the convergence of science and Buddhism and the other great contemplative traditions of the world, we may reintegrate these noblest of pursuits and help to heal our world from its current state of disintegration, alienation, conflict, and suffering.

NOTES

1. PRINCIPLES OF CONTEMPLATIVE SCIENCE

1. Josef Pieper, *Happiness and Contemplation*, trans. Richard and Clara Winston (Chicago: Henry Regnery, 1966), 73.
2. Ibid., 73–74.
3. Aristotle, *Nicomachean Ethics*, trans. Terence Irwin (Indianapolis: Hackett, 1985), 1098a16.
4. Augustine, *Letters 100–155* (*Epistolae*), trans. Roland Teske (Hyde Park, NY: New City Press, 2003), 118, 13.
5. Augustine, *The Confessions*, trans. Maria Boulding (Hyde Park, NY: New City Press, 1997), 33.
6. His Holiness the Dalai Lama and Howard C. Cutler, M.D., *The Art of Happiness: A Handbook for Living* (New York: Riverhead, 1998), 15.
7. Joseph Maréchal, S.J., *Studies in the Psychology of the Mystics*, trans. Algar Thorold (London: Burns Oates & Washbourne, 1927), 101.
8. Śāntideva, *A Guide to the Bodhisattva Way of Life*, trans. Vesna A. Wallace and B. Alan Wallace (Ithaca, NY: Snow Lion, 1997), IX:1.
9. John Burnaby, *Amor Dei: A Study of the Religion of St. Augustine* (Norwich, England: The Canterbury Press, 1991), 107.
10. Ibid., 104.
11. Paul Ekman, Richard J. Davidson, Matthieu Ricard, and B. Alan Wallace, "Buddhist and Psychological Perspectives on Emotions and Well-Being," *Current Directions in Psychological Science* 14, no. 2 (2005): 59–63.
12. Tim Kasser, *The High Price of Materialism* (Boston: MIT Press, 2002), 22.
13. H. L. Bond, trans., *Nicholas of Cusa: Selected Spiritual Writings* (New York: Paulist Press, 1997), 242.
14. Śāntideva, *A Guide to the Bodhisattva Way of Life*, I:28.

15. Ibid., VIII:1.
16. Kallistos Ware, "Ways of Prayer and Contemplation: I. Eastern," in *Christian Spirituality: Origins to the Twelfth Century*, ed. Bernard McGinn and John Meyendorff (New York: Crossroad, 1985), 398.
17. Maréchal, *Studies in the Psychology of the Mystics*, 168.
18. *Udāna* 1, 10.
19. Plato, *Phaedo*, in *The Collected Dialogues of Plato*, ed. Edith Hamilton and Huntington Cairns, trans. Hugh Tredennick (Princeton: Princeton University Press, Bollingen Series LXXI, 1961), 80–82.
20. Ibid., 81a.
21. Ibid., 81c–d.
22. Ware, "Ways of Prayer and Contemplation: I. Eastern," 397.
23. Augustine, *The Free Choice of the Will*, trans. Francis E. Tourscher (Philadelphia: Peter Reilly, 1937), book III, chs. 20–21.
24. Ibid., 379.
25. William James, *Essays in Religion and Morality* (Cambridge, MA: Harvard University Press, 1989), 85–86.
26. Ibid., 87.
27. For a partial list of his articles published in scientific journals, see: http://www.healthsystem.virginia.edu/internet/personalitystudies/publications.cfm.
28. See also Pim van Lommel, Ruud van Wees, Vincent Meyers, and Ingrid Elfferich, "Near-Death Experience in Survivors of Cardiac Arrest: A Prospective Study in the Netherlands," *The Lancet* 358 (2001): 2039–45.
29. Richard P. Feynman, *The Character of Physical Law* (Cambridge, MA: MIT Press, 1983), 158.
30. John R. Searle, *Consciousness and Language* (Cambridge, England: Cambridge University Press, 2002), 18.
31. David J. Chalmers, *Conscious Mind: In Search of a Fundamental Theory* (New York: Oxford University Press, 1996).
32. William James, *The Principles of Psychology* (New York: Dover, 1950), I:191–92.
33. B. Alan Wallace, *The Attention Revolution: Unlocking the Power of the Focused Mind* (Boston: Wisdom, 2006).
34. For a detailed explanation of this theory, see B. Alan Wallace, *Choosing Reality: A Buddhist View of Physics and the Mind* (Ithaca, NY: Snow Lion, 1996), 180–90.
35. Düdjom Lingpa, *The Vajra Essence: From the Matrix of Pure Appearances and Primordial Consciousness, a Tantra on the Self-originating Nature of Existence*, trans. B. Alan Wallace (Alameda, CA: Mirror of Wisdom, 2004), 92.
36. Anne C. Klein, "Mental Concentration and the Unconditioned: A Buddhist Case for Unmediated Experience," in *Paths to Liberation: The Mārga and Its Transformations in Buddhist Thought*, ed. Robert E. Buswell Jr. and Robert M. Gimello (Honolulu: University of Hawaii Press, 1992), 278, 294.
37. Düdjom Lingpa, *The Vajra Essence*, 30.
38. Henning Genz, *Nothingness: The Science of Empty Space* (Cambridge, MA: Perseus, 1999), 26.

39. Russell Targ, *Limitless Mind: A Guide to Remote Viewing and Transformation of Consciousness* (Novato, CA: New World Library, 2004).

40. Genz, *Nothingness*, 261.

41. K. C. Cole, *The Hole in the Universe: How Scientists Peered Over the Edge of Emptiness and Found Everything* (New York: Harcourt, 2001), 236.

42. Genz, *Nothingness*, 312.

43. Cole, *The Hole in the Universe*, 177–78.

44. H. H. the Dalai Lama, *Dzogchen: The Heart Essence of the Great Perfection*, trans. Geshe Thupten Jinpa and Richard Barron (Ithaca, NY: Snow Lion, 2000), 48–49.

45. Antonio Damasio, *The Feeling of What Happens: Body and Emotion in the Making of Consciousness* (New York: Harcourt, 1999), 28.

46. Daniel J. Boorstin, *The Discoverers: A History of Man's Search to Know His World and Himself* (New York: Vintage, 1985), xv.

47. Cole, *The Hole in the Universe*, 235.

48. Ware, "Ways of Prayer and Contemplation: I. Eastern," 399.

49. Ibid., 237.

50. Ibid., 238.

51. Bond, trans., *Nicholas of Cusa*, 246.

52. Dom Cuthbert Butler, *Western Mysticism: The Teaching of Augustine, Gregory, and Bernard on Contemplation and the Contemplative Life*, 3rd ed. (London: Constable, 1967), 49.

53. Bond, trans., *Nicholas of Cusa*, 263.

54. Ibid., 238.

55. Ibid., 261.

56. Thomas Aquinas, *Sentences* of Peter Lombard 4d. 26, 1, 2. Cited in Pieper, *Happiness and Contemplation*, 96.

57. Thomas Aquinas, *Commentary on Aristotle's Nicomachean Ethics* 10, 11; no. 2101. Cited in Pieper, *Happiness and Contemplation*, 94.

2. WHERE SCIENCE AND RELIGION COLLIDE

1. Aleksandr Oparin, *The Origin of Life*, trans. Sergius Morgulis (New York: Macmillan, 1938).

2. Edward O. Wilson, *Consilience: The Unity of Knowledge* (New York: Knopf, 1998), 60.

3. Richard P. Feynman, R. B. Leighton, and M. Sands, *The Feynman Lectures on Physics* (Reading, MA: Addison-Wesley, 1963), 1–9.

4. Richard Dawkins, *The Selfish Gene* (New York: Oxford University Press, 1978), 56.

5. Antonio Damasio, *The Feeling of What Happens: Body and Emotion in the Making of Consciousness* (New York: Harcourt, 1999), 322.

6. Richard Dawkins, *The Blind Watchmaker* (New York: Norton, 1987), 5.

7. Steven Weinberg, *The First Three Minutes: A Modern View of the Origin of the Universe* (New York: Basic Books, 1988), 154.

8. Cited in Arthur Koestler, *The Ghost in the Machine* (New York: Macmillan, 1967), 5.

9. Werner Heisenberg, *Physics and Philosophy: The Revolution in Modern Science* (New York: Harper and Row, 1962), 58.

10. Cited in Werner Heisenberg, *Physics and Beyond: Encounters and Conversations* (New York: Harper and Row, 1971), 63.

11. Dawkins, *The Selfish Gene*, 207.

12. Wilson, *Consilience*, 115.

13. Ibid., 261.

14. Ibid., 110.

15. Brian Greene, *The Elegant Universe: Superstrings, Hidden Dimensions, and the Quest for the Ultimate Theory* (New York: Norton, 1999).

16. Cited in K. C. Cole, "In Patterns, Not Particles, Physicists Trust," *Los Angeles Times*, March 4, 1999.

17. Richard P. Feynman, R. B. Leighton, and M. Sands, *The Feynman Lectures on Physics* (Cambridge, MA: MIT Press, 1965), sec. 4–2.

18. WorldNetDaily, February 27, 2003, http://www.worldnetdaily.com/news/article.asp?ARTICLE_ID=31266. The data poll was collected by Harris Poll from January 21 to 27. 2,201 subjects. Margin of error 2%.

19. Source: http://www.vision.org/trdl/2000/trdl000123.html.

20. Edward J. Larson and Larry Witham, "Leading Scientists Still Reject God," *Nature* 394 (1998): 313.

21. Wilson, *Consilience*, 238.

22. Cf. B. Alan Wallace, *The Taboo of Subjectivity: Toward a New Science of Consciousness* (New York: Oxford University Press, 2000).

23. William James, *A Pluralistic Universe* (Cambridge, MA: Harvard University Press, 1977), 142.

3. THE STUDY OF CONSCIOUSNESS, EAST AND WEST

An earlier version of this essay was published under the title "A Science of Consciousness: Buddhism (1), the Modern West (0)" in *The Pacific World: Journal of the Institute of Buddhist Studies*, 3rd series, no. 4 (Fall 2002): 15–31.

1. Plato, *Phaedo,* trans. Robin Waterfield. (New York: Oxford University Press, 2002), 230A.

2. John R. Searle, *The Rediscovery of the Mind* (Cambridge, MA: MIT Press, 1994), 79.

3. Stephen LaBerge, "Lucid Dreaming and the Yoga of the Dream State: A Psychophysiological Perspective, in *Buddhism and Science: Breaking New Ground,* ed. B. Alan Wallace (New York: Columbia University Press, 2003), 233–58.

4. Searle, *The Rediscovery of the Mind*, 97.

5. See, for example, Daniel C. Matt, "*Ayin*: The Concept of Nothingness in Jewish Mysticism," in *The Problem of Pure Consciousness: Mysticism and Philosophy*, ed. Robert K. C. Forman (New York: Oxford University Press, 1990); *The Essential Kabbalah: The Heart of Jewish Mysticism* (San Francisco: HarperSanFrancisco, 1995).

6. Owen Chadwick, trans. and ed., *The Conferences of Cassian in Western Asceticism* (Philadelphia: Westminster Press, 1958).

7. Dom Cuthbert Butler, *Western Mysticism: The Teaching of Augustine, Gregory, and Bernard on Contemplation and the Contemplative Life*, 3rd ed. (London: Constable, 1967), 26.

8. John Burnaby, *Amor Dei: A Study of the Religion of St. Augustine* (1938; reprint, Norwich: Canterbury Press, 1991), 52, 67.

9. M. O. C. Walshe, trans., *Meister Eckhart: Sermons and Treatises*, Vols. I–III (Longmead: Element Books, 1979), 1:7.

10. Exodus 22:18. *New International Version* (Grand Rapids, MI: Zondervan Bible Publishers, 1984).

11. John B. Watson, *Behaviorism* (1913; reprint, New York: Norton, 1970).

12. Antonio R. Damasio, "How the Brain Creates the Mind," *Scientific American* 12, no. 1 (2002): 4–9.

13. Edward O. Wilson, *Consilience: The Unity of Knowledge* (New York: Knopf, 1998), 96–97.

14. Daniel Dennett, *Consciousness Explained* (Boston: Little, Brown, 1991), 21–22.

15. Searle, *The Rediscovery of the Mind*, 247.

16. Wilson, *Consilience*, 60–61.

17. Ibid., 60.

18. F. Crick and C. Koch, "Towards a Neurobiological Theory of Consciousness," in *The Nature of Consciousness: Philosophical Debates*, ed. N. Block, O. Flanagan, and G. Güzeldere (Cambridge, MA: MIT Press, 1998), 277–92.

19. William James, *The Principles of Psychology* (1890; reprint, New York: Dover, 1950), I:185.

20. Ibid., I:416–24.

21. Ibid., I:424.

22. One very promising development in modern psychology in this regard is the emergence of "positive psychology." See C. R. Snyder and Shane J. Lopez, eds., *Handbook of Positive Psychology* (New York: Oxford University Press, 2002).

23. For a more detailed presentation of these Four Noble Truths within a contemporary context, see B. Alan Wallace, *Balancing the Mind: A Tibetan Buddhist Approach to Refining Attention* (Ithaca, NY: Snow Lion, 2005).

24. For a detailed account of this type of attentional training, see B. Alan Wallace, *Balancing the Mind* and *The Attention Revolution: Unlocking the Power of the Focused Mind* (Boston: Wisdom, 2006).

25. Kamalaśīla, *First Bhāvanākrama*, ed. G. Tucci, in *Minor Buddhist Texts, Part II* (Rome: Istituto italiano per il Medio ed Estremo Oriente, 1958), 205.

26. Wallace, *Balancing the Mind*, 118.

27. For a lucid presentation of Buddhist ethics presented within a modern, secular context, see H. H. the Dalai Lama, *Ethics for the New Millennium* (New York: Riverhead, 1999).

28. Aristotle, *Nicomachean Ethics*, trans. Terence Irwin (Indianapolis: Hackett, 1985).

29. For a discussion of scholasticism within Indo-Tibetan Buddhism, see José Ignacio Cabezón, *Buddhism and Language: A Study of Indo-Tibetan Scholasticism* (Albany: State University of New York Press, 1994).

30. See Robert H. Sharf, "Buddhist Modernism and the Rhetoric of Meditative Experiences," *Numen* 42 (1995): 228–83; "Experience," in *Critical Terms for Religious Studies*, ed. Mark C. Taylor (Chicago: University of Chicago Press, 1998), 94–116.

31. Personal communication from Geshe Thupten Jinpa, June 6, 2002.

32. Antonio R. Damasio, *The Feeling of What Happens: Body and Emotion in the Making of Consciousness* (New York: Harcourt, 1999), 9. See also Searle, *The Rediscovery of the Mind*, 100.

33. Daniel J. Boorstin, *The Discoverers: A History of Man's Search to Know His World and Himself* (New York: Vintage, 1985), xv.

4. SPIRITUAL AWAKENING AND OBJECTIVE KNOWLEDGE

1. *Catuḥśataka*, vs. 276. See Ruth Sonam, trans., *Yogic Deeds of Bodhisattvas: Gyeltsap on Āryadeva's Four Hundred*, commentary by Geshe Sonam Rinchen (Ithaca, NY: Snow Lion, 1994), 239–40.

2. R. Chene, "Is Every Mediation Multicultural?" in conference handbook, Northern California Mediation Association, March 18, 2000, 36.

3. T. Tillemans, "Indian and Tibetan Mādhyamikas on *mānasapratyakṣa*," *Tibet Journal* 14, no. 1 (1989): 70–85.

4. Anne C. Klein, *Path to the Middle: Oral Mādhyamika Philosophy in Tibet* (Albany: State University of New York Press, 1994), 278, 294; B. Alan Wallace, *Balancing the Mind: A Tibetan Buddhist Approach to Refining Attention* (Ithaca, NY: Snow Lion, 2005), 230–43.

5. Lawrence Bond, *On Nicholas of Cusa: Selected Spiritual Writings* (New York: Paulist Press, 1997), 254–5.

6. B. Alan Wallace, *The Taboo of Subjectivity: Toward a New Science of Consciousness* (New York: Oxford University Press, 2000), 41–56.

7. B. Alan Wallace, *Choosing Reality: A Buddhist View of Physics and the Mind* (Ithaca, NY: Snow Lion, 1996), 62.

8. Thomas Nagel, *The View from Nowhere* (New York: Oxford University Press, 1986).

9. Edward O. Wilson, *Consilience: The Unity of Knowledge* (New York: Knopf, 1998), 160.

10. Ibid., 163.

11. Paul C. W. Davies, "An Overview of the Contributions of John Archibald Wheeler," in *Science and Ultimate Reality: Quantum Theory, Cosmology and Complexity, Honoring John Wheeler's 90th Birthday*, ed. John D. Barrow, Paul C. W. Davies, and Charles L. Harper Jr. (Cambridge: Cambridge University Press, 2004), 3–26.

12. Sigmund Freud, *Civilization and Its Discontents*, trans. and ed. James Strachey (New York: Norton, 1961), 16.

13. E. Schrödinger, *Mind and Matter* (Cambridge: Cambridge University Press, 1958).

14. John R. Searle, *The Rediscovery of the Mind* (Cambridge, MA: MIT Press, 1994), 95.

15. Wilson, *Consilience*, 37.

16. Ibid., 97.

17. Ibid.

18. K. Danziger, "The History of Introspection Reconsidered," *Journal of the History of the Behavioral Sciences* 16 (1980): 241–62.

19. Wilson, *Consilience*, 110.

20. Immanuel Kant, *Metaphysical Foundations of Natural Science*, trans. James Ellington (1786; reprint, Indianapolis: Bobbs-Merrill, 1970), 8.

21. Peter Harvey, *The Selfless Mind: Personality, Consciousness and Nirvana in Early Buddhism* (Surrey, England: Curzon Press, 1995), 79.

22. Ibid., 82.

23. B. Ñāṇamoli, *The Life of the Buddha According to the Pali Canon* (Kandy, Sri Lanka: Buddhist Publication Society, 1992), 10–29.

24. Ibid., 24.

25. Ibid.

26. Ibid., 25.

27. B. Alan Wallace, "The Buddhist Tradition of Śamatha: Methods for Refining and Examining Consciousness," *Journal of Consciousness Studies* 6, no. 2–3 (1999): 175–87.

28. Nyanaponika Thera, *The Heart of Buddhist Meditation* (New York: Samuel Weiser, 1973).

29. Ibid., 59.

30. Stephen Batchelor, *Buddhism Without Beliefs: A Contemporary Guide to Awakening* (New York: Riverhead, 1997), 5.

31. R. H. Sharf, "Experience," in *Critical Terms for Religious Studies*, ed. Mark C. Taylor (Chicago: University of Chicago Press, 1998), 102.

32. Ibid., 99.

33. Ibid.

34. G. C. C. Chang, trans. and ed., *The Hundred Thousand Songs of Milarepa* (Boulder, CO: Shambhala Publications, 1962).

35. R. H. Sharf, "Buddhist Modernism and the Rhetoric of Meditative Experiences," *Numen* 42 (1995): 228–83.

36. Ibid., 108–9.

37. Ibid., 110.

38. L. Gómez, "Measuring the Immeasurable: Reflections on Unreasonable Reasoning," in *Buddhist Theology: Critical Reflections by Contemporary Buddhist Scholars*, ed. Roger R. Jackson and John Makransky (Surrey, England: Curzon, 1999), 371.

39. Sharf, "Buddhist Modernism and the Rhetoric of Meditative Experiences," 99.

40. Ibid., 114.

41. Wallace, *The Taboo of Subjectivity*, 75–120.

42. Wallace, *Balancing the Mind*.

43. Ruth Sonam, *Atisha's Lamp for the Path*, commentary by Geshe Sonam Rinchen (Ithaca, NY: Snow Lion, 1997), 89–105.

44. William James, *The Principles of Psychology* (1890; reprint, New York: Dover, 1950), I:185.

45. B.G. Dreyfus, *Recognizing Reality: Dharmakīrti's Philosophy and Its Tibetan Interpretations* (Delhi: Sri Satguru, 1997), 349–50; Gendün-drup (dge 'dun grub), *Ornament of Reasoning, a Great Treatise on Valid Cognition (tshad ma'i bstan bcos chen po rigs pa'i rgyan)* (Mundgod, India: Loling Press, 1985), 38.3-.10.

46. Tsongkhapa, *The Great Treatise on the Stages of the Path to Enlightenment*, vol. 3 (Ithaca, NY: Snow Lion, 2002), 178.

47. Dreyfus, *Recognizing Reality*, 285–315.

48. B. Van Fraassen, *The Empirical Stance* (New Haven: Yale University Press, 2002).

49. J. Bronkhorst, *Why Is There Philosophy in India* (Amsterdam: Royal Netherlands Academy of Arts and Sciences, 1999), 6.

50. Wallace, *The Taboo of Subjectivity*, 145–75.

51. Walpola Rahula, *What the Buddha Taught* (New York: Grove Weidenfeld, 1974), 2–3.

52. D. Shastri, *Tattvasaṃgraha* (Varanasi: Bauddhabharati, 1968), 3587.

53. R. Gnoli, ed., *The Pramāṇavārttikam of Dharmakīrti* (Rome: Serie Orientale Roma 23, 1960), 22.

54. William James, "A World of Pure Experience," in *The Writings of William James*, ed. John J. McDermott (1912; reprint, Chicago: University of Chicago Press, 1977), 194–214.

55. Wilson, *Consilience*, 59.

56. Wallace, *Choosing Reality*, 52, 85–86; Wallace, *The Taboo of Subjectivity*, 68–69; Davies, "An Overview of the Contributions of John Archibald Wheeler," 17.

57. Dreyfus, *Recognizing Reality*, 416–27.

58. Roger R. Jackson, *Is Enlightenment Possible?: Dharmakīrti and rGyal tshab rje on Knowledge, Rebirth, No-self and Liberation* (Ithaca, NY: Snow Lion, 1993).

59. Roger R. Jackson, "In Search of a Postmodern Middle," in *Buddhist Theology: Critical Reflections by Contemporary Buddhist Scholars*, ed. Roger R. Jackson and John Makransky (Surrey, England: Curzon, 1999), 236.

60. T. Tillemans, *Scripture, Logic, Language: Essays on Dharmakīrti and His Tibetan Successors* (Boston: Wisdom, 1999), 29–30.

61. H. H. the Dalai Lama, *The Universe in a Single Atom: The Convergence of Science and Spirituality* (New York: Morgan Road, 2005), 28–29.

62. Tillemans, *Scripture, Logic, Language*, 30.

63. Ibid., 41.

5. BUDDHIST NONTHEISM, POLYTHEISM, AND MONOTHEISM

1. Paul Williams, "Out of My Head," *The Tablet* (Aug. 5, 2000):1046.

2. Stephen Batchelor, *Buddhism Without Beliefs: A Contemporary Guide to Awakening* (New York: Riverhead, 1997), 15–18, 36, 114–15.

3. *Pāṭika Sutta* 2.14–20.

4. H. H. the Dalai Lama, *The Universe in a Single Atom: The Convergence of Science and Spirituality* (New York: Morgan Road, 2005), 90–92.

5. Peter Harvey, *The Selfless Mind: Personality, Consciousness, and Nirvana in Early Buddhism* (Surrey, England: Curzon, 1995), 160.

6. *Aṅguttara Nikāya* A.I.9–10.

7. *Aṅguttara Nikāya* A.I.10–11.

8. Paravahera Vajirañāṇa, *Buddhist Meditation in Theory and Practice* (Kuala Lumpur, Malaysia: Buddhist Missionary Society, 1975), 151; cf. Buddhaghosa, *Visuddhimagga* IV.33.

9. Harvey, *The Selfless Mind*, 159.

10. *Milindapañha*, 299–300.

11. *Kathāvatthu* 615.

12. For an excellent overview of Theravāda, Mahāyāna, and Vajrayāna Buddhism, see B. Peter Harvey, *An Introduction to Buddhism: Teachings, History, and Practices* (Cambridge: Cambridge University Press, 1990).

13. *Cūla-Māluṅkyaputta-sutta* 63.

14. *Milindapañha* 73.

15. R. H. Robinson, *The Buddhist Religion* (Belmont, CA: Dickenson, 1970), 38–39.

16. Harvey, *The Selfless Mind*, 98–101.

17. Śāntideva, *A Guide to the Bodhisattva Way of Life*, trans. Vesna A. Wallace and B. Alan Wallace (Ithaca, NY: Snow Lion, 1997), IX:118–25.

18. Cited in Harvey, *The Selfless Mind*, 175.

19. *Laṅkāvatāra Sūtra*, 77.

20. *Laṅkāvatāra Sūtra*, 220.

21. Cited in Paul Williams, *Mahāyāna Buddhism: The Doctrinal Foundations* (London: Routledge, 1989), 98.

22. Cited in ibid., 99.

23. *Ratnagotra-vibhāga*, vv. 51, 84.

24. *Ratnagotra-vibhāga*, v. 149.

25. Harvey, *The Selfless Mind*, 176.

26. Alex and Hideko Wayman, trans., *The Lion's Road of Queen Śrīmālā* (Delhi: Motilal Banarsidass, 1990), 98.

27. K. H. Holmes and K. Holmes, *The Changeless Continuity*, 2nd ed. (Eskdalemuir, Scotland: Karma Drubgyud Darjay Ling, 1985), 72–73.

28. Thich Nhat Hanh, *Living Buddha, Living Christ* (New York: Riverhead, 1997).

29. *Vimalaprabhā* II:168–70.

30. *Vimalaprabhā* II:169.

31. *Kālacakratantra*, V 65.

32. Düdjom Lingpa, *The Vajra Essence: From the Matrix of Pure Appearances and Primordial Consciousness, a Tantra on the Self-Originating Nature of Existence*, trans. B. Alan Wallace (Alameda, CA: Mirror of Wisdom, 2004).

33. Ibid., 90.

34. Ibid., 80.

35. Padmasambhava, *Natural Liberation: Padmasambhava's Teachings on the Six*

Bardos, commentary by Gyatrul Rinpoche; trans. B. Alan Wallace (Boston: Wisdom, 1998), 122.

36. Donald F. Duclow, "Divine Nothingness and Self-Creation in John Scotus Eriugena," *The Journal of Religion* 57, no. 2 (April 1977): 110.

37. John Scotus Eriugena, *Periphyseon (De divisione naturae)*, ed. H. J. Floss, Migne *Patrologia latina* 122, 680D–81A, trans. Donald F. Duclow (Ridgewood, NJ: Gregg Press, 1965), 110. Cf. *Bodhicāryāvatāra* IX:2. "This truth is recognized as being of two kinds: conventional and ultimate. Ultimate reality is beyond the scope of the intellect. The intellect is called conventional reality."

38. Cited in Śāntideva, *Śikṣā-samuccaya*, trans. Cecil Bendall and W. H. D. Rouse (Delhi: Motilal Banarsidass, 1981), 220–21. See also Thomas Tomasic, "Negative Theology and Subjectivity: An Approach to the Tradition of the Pseudo-Dionysius," *International Philosophical Quarterly* 9 (1969).

39. H. Lawrence Bond, *On Nicholas of Cusa: Selected Spiritual Writings* (New York: Paulist Press, 1997), 225.

40. Ibid., 223.

41. Ibid. 230–31.

42. Cited in Karma Chagmé, *A Spacious Path to Freedom*, trans. B. Alan Wallace (Ithaca, NY: Snow Lion, 1998), 107; cf. W. Y. Evans-Wentz, ed., *The Tibetan Book of the Great Liberation* (London: Oxford University Press, 1968), 208–9.

43. Aldous Huxley, *The Perennial Philosophy* (London: Chatto & Windus, 1946).

44. William James, *The Varieties of Religious Experience: A Study in Human Nature* (New York: Longmans, Green, 1902), 428.

6. WORLDS OF INTERSUBJECTIVITY

This essay was first published under the title "Intersubjectivity in Indo-Tibetan Buddhism" in *Journal of Consciousness Studies* 8, no. 5–7 (2001): 209–30.

1. A detailed discussion of all five of these systems of meditation is presented in B. Alan Wallace, *Genuine Happiness: Meditation as the Path to Fulfillment* (Hoboken, NJ: Wiley, 2005).

2. For a more elaborate discussion of meditative quiescence and its relation to contemplative insight, see Tsongkhapa, *The Great Treatise on the Stages of the Path to Enlightenment* (Ithaca, NY: Snow Lion, 2002), 3:13–26; B. Alan Wallace, *Balancing the Mind: A Tibetan Buddhist Approach to Refining Attention* (Ithaca, NY: Snow Lion, 2005) and *The Attention Revolution: Unlocking the Power of the Focused Mind* (Boston: Wisdom, 2006).

3. *Aṅguttara Nikāya* V, 201ff.

4. Paravahera Vajirañāṇa, *Buddhist Meditation in Theory and Practice*, 249.

5. Peter Harvey, *The Selfless Mind*, 160.

6. See Paravahera Vajirañāṇa, *Buddhist Meditation in Theory and Practice* (Kuala Lumpur, Malaysia: Buddhist Missionary Society, 1975), 151, 327–28, David J. Kalupahana, *The Principles of Buddhist Psychology* (Albany: State University of New York Press, 1987), 112–15, and *Aṅguttara Nikāya* A.I.9–10, A.I.61.

7. *Aṅguttara Nikāya* A.I.10–11.

8. See the section "Quiescence According to Mahāmudrā and Atiyoga" in Wallace, *Balancing the Mind*; James Haughton Woods, *The Yoga System of Patañjali* (Delhi: Motilal Banarsidass, 1983); and Robert K. C. Forman, ed., *The Problem of Pure Consciousness: Mysticism and Philosophy* (New York: Oxford University Press, 1990).

9. Soma Thera, *The Way of Mindfulness: The Satipaṭṭhāna Sutta and Commentary* (Kandy, Sri Lanka: Buddhist Publication Society, 1975); R. M. L. Gethin, *The Buddhist Path to Awakening* (Oxford: Oneworld, 2001), 29–68.

10. *Udāna* 8.

11. Thera, *Satipaṭṭhānasutta*, 5.

12. For a discussion of observing the four subjects of mindfulness inwardly, outwardly, and both inwardly and outwardly, see Nyanaponika Thera, *The Heart of Buddhist Meditation* (New York: Samuel Weiser, 1973), 58–60.

13. William James, *The Principles of Psychology* (1890; reprint, New York: Dover, 1950), 322.

14. Ibid., 290–91.

15. William James, "A World of Pure Experience," in *The Writings of William James: A Comprehensive Edition*, ed. John J. McDermott (Chicago: University of Chicago Press, 1977), 195.

16. *Milindapañha* 37–38.

17. Buddhaghosa, *Visuddhimagga*, I:IX; Harvey B. Aronson, *Love and Sympathy in Theravāda Buddhism* (Delhi: Motilal Banarsidass, 1980); B. Alan Wallace, *The Four Immeasurables: Cultivating a Boundless Heart*, rev. ed. (Ithaca, NY: Snow Lion, 2004).

18. Martin Buber, *I and Thou*, trans. Walter Kaufmann (1937; reprint, New York: Touchstone, 1996).

19. *Udāna* 47.

20. For a fascinating account of a cross-cultural dialogue with the Dalai Lama on this theme, see Daniel Goleman, ed., *Healing Emotions: Conversations with the Dalai Lama on Mindfulness, Emotions, and Health* (Boston: Shambhala, 1997), 189–207.

21. B. Alan Wallace, *Buddhism with an Attitude: The Tibetan Seven-Point Mind-Training* (Ithaca, NY: Snow Lion, 2001), 154–63.

22. Śāntideva, *A Guide to the Bodhisattva Way of Life*, trans. Vesna A. Wallace and B. Alan Wallace (Ithaca, NY: Snow Lion, 1997), VIII:94.

23. Jay L. Garfield, trans., *The Fundamental Wisdom of the Middle Way: Nāgārjuna's Mūlamadhyamakakārikā* (New York: Oxford University Press, 1995).

24. Glenn H. Mullin, trans., *Tsongkhapa's Six Yogas of Naropa* (Ithaca, NY: Snow Lion, 1996), 174.

25. Cf. Paul C. W. Davies, "An Overview of the Contributions of John Archibald Wheeler," in *Science and Ultimate Reality: Quantum Theory, Cosmology and Complexity, Honoring John Wheeler's 90th Birthday*, ed. John D. Barrow, Paul C. W. Davies, and Charles L. Harper Jr. (Cambridge: Cambridge University Press, 2004), 8–10.

26. This definition is taken from Hilary Putnam, *Realism with a Human Face*, ed. James Conant (Cambridge, MA: Harvard University Press, 1990), 30.

27. Ibid., 28.

28. Hilary Putnam, "Replies and Comments," *Erkenntnis* 34, no. 3 (1991): 407. I have discussed this point at greater length in the chapter "The World of Human Experience" in B. Alan Wallace, *The Taboo of Subjectivity: Toward a New Science of Consciousness* (New York: Oxford University Press, 2000).

29. Traditional Tibetan Buddhist accounts of the practice of dream yoga can be found in Padmasambhava, *Natural Liberation: Padmasambhava's Teachings on the Six Bardos*, commentary by Gyatrul Rinpoche; trans. B. Alan Wallace (Boston: Wisdom, 1998), part 2, ch. 4, and Mullin, *Tsongkhapa's Six Yogas of Naropa*, 172–84.

30. For a clear, modern account of the theory and practice of lucid dreaming, see Stephen LaBerge and Howard Rheingold, *Exploring the World of Lucid Dreaming* (New York: Ballantine, 1990).

31. This same point is made regarding one's realization of emptiness during the waking state in Śāntideva, *A Guide to the Bodhisattva Way of Life*, IX:30–32.

32. Padmasambhava, *Natural Liberation*, 164.

33. Ibid., 168.

34. Detailed, traditional presentations of this mode of investigation are found in the "Insight" chapter in Padmasambhava, *Natural Liberation*, and the "Insight" chapter of the seventeenth-century classic by Karma Chagmé, *A Spacious Path to Freedom: Practical Instructions on the Union of Mahāmudrā and Atiyoga*, commentary by Gyatrul Rinpoche; trans. B. Alan Wallace (Ithaca, NY: Snow Lion, 1998).

35. Padmasambhava, *Natural Liberation*, 116.

36. Ibid., 108.

7. *ŚAMATHA*: THE CONTEMPLATIVE REFINEMENT OF ATTENTION

This essay was first published under the title "The Buddhist Tradition of *Śamatha*: Methods for Refining and Examining Consciousness" in *Journal of Consciousness Studies* 6, no. 2–3 (1999): 175–87. For more extensive information, please see B. Alan Wallace, *The Attention Revolution: Unlocking the Power of the Focused Mind* (Boston: Wisdom, 2006).

1. *Ratnameghasūtra*, cited in Śāntideva's *Śikṣāsamuccaya*, ed. P. D. Vaidya (Darbhanga: Mithila Institute, 1961), 68. This passage is found in the English translation of Śāntideva's work by Cecil Bendall and W. H. D. Rouse (Delhi: Motilal Banarsidass, 1981), 121. A similar point is made by the Buddha in the opening verse of *The Dhammapada*: "All phenomena are preceded by the mind, issue forth from the mind, and consist of the mind" (*The Dhammapada*, ed. Nikunja Vihari Banerjee [New Delhi: Munshiram Manoharlal, 1989], ch. 1, v. 1).

2. B. Alan Wallace, *Balancing the Mind: A Tibetan Buddhist Approach to Refining Attention* (Ithaca, NY: Snow Lion, 2005), 168. A mental process is said to be *intentional* not because one intends for it to occur, but because it has its own cognized object or objects.

3. Compulsive desire is a mental affliction that by its very nature superimposes a quality of attractiveness upon its object and yearns for it. It distorts the cognition of that object, for attachment exaggerates admirable qualities and screens out disagreeable qualities. Cf. Herbert V. Guenther and Leslie S. Kawamura, *Mind in Buddhist Psychology* (Emeryville: Dharma Publishing, 1975), 96; Geshe Rabten, *The Mind and Its Functions*, trans. Stephen Batchelor (Mt. Pèlerin, Switz.: Tharpa Choeling, 1979), 74–75.

4. Vasubandhu, *Abhidharmakośabhāṣyam*, French trans. Louis de La Vallée Poussin; English trans. Leo M. Pruden (Berkeley: Asian Humanities Press, 1991), 2:474. Cf. Jamgön Kongtrul Lodrö Tayé, *Myriad Worlds: Buddhist Cosmology in Abhidharma, Kālacakra, and Dzog-chen*, trans. and ed. International Translation Committee (Ithaca, NY: Snow Lion, 1995), 168–69.

5. For a detailed account of nonascertaining cognition, see Lati Rinbochay, *Mind in Tibetan Buddhism*, trans. and ed. Elizabeth Napper (Valois: Gabriel/Snow Lion, 1981), 92–110.

6. The technique of focusing on a pebble or stick is found in the section entitled "Instructions on Quiescence with Signs" in *Natural Liberation: Padmasambhava's Teachings on the Six Bardos*, commentary by Gyaltrul Rinpoche; trans. B. Alan Wallace (Boston: Wisdom, 1998), 95–96. Tsongkhapa opts for focusing on an image of the Buddha in *The Great Treatise on the Stages of the Path to Enlightenment* (Ithaca, NY: Snow Lion, 2002), 3:42–46. For a clear discussion of the technique of focusing on a Buddha image by a contemporary Tibetan contemplative, see Gen Lamrimpa, *Calming the Mind: Tibetan Buddhist Teachings on the Cultivation of Meditative Quiescence*, trans. B. Alan Wallace (Ithaca, NY: Snow Lion, 1995).

7. Cf. Jeffrey Hopkins, *Meditation on Emptiness* (London: Wisdom, 1983), 232–34.

8. Śāntideva, *A Guide to the Bodhisattva Way of Life*, trans. Vesna A. Wallace and B. Alan Wallace (Ithaca, NY: Snow Lion, 1997), V:108.

9. Intelligence is defined as a mental process having the unique function of differentiating specific attributes or faults and merits of objects that are maintained with mindfulness. Cf. Geshe Rabten, *The Mind and Its Functions*, 63.

10. Vasubandhu, *Abhidharmakośabhāṣyam*, 1:206, 272.

11. *Ratnacūḍasūtra*, cited in Śāntideva, *Śikṣa-samuccaya: A Compendium of Buddhist Doctrine*, ed. P. D. Vaidya (Darbhanga, India: Mithila Institute, 1961), 220–21.

12. Śāntideva, *A Guide to the Bodhisattva Way of Life*, IX:23. Cf. H. H. the Dalai Lama, *Transcendent Wisdom: A Teaching on the Wisdom Section of Shantideva's Guide to the Bodhisattva Way of Life*, trans., ed., and annot. B. Alan Wallace (Ithaca, NY: Snow Lion, 1994), 26–31.

13. Cf. M. I. Posner, *Chronometric Exploration of Mind* (Hillsdale, NJ: Lawrence Erlbaum Associates, 1978).

14. William James, *The Principles of Psychology* (1890; reprint, New York: Dover, 1950), I:420.

15. This topic is discussed in the section entitled "Identifying the Will and the Means of Stopping Laxity and Excitation" in Wallace, *Balancing the Mind*.

16. James, *The Principles of Psychology*, I:423.

17. William James, *Talks to Teachers: On Psychology; and to Students on Some of Life's Ideals* (1899; reprint, New York: Norton, 1958), 78.

18. James, *The Principles of Psychology*, I:425.

19. Hopkins, *Meditation on Emptiness*, 233.

20. A clear discussion of this technique is found in the section entitled "The Cultivation of Attention" in Karma Chagmé, *A Spacious Path to Freedom: Practical Instructions on the Union of Mahāmudrā and Atiyoga*, commentary by Gyatrul Rinpoche; trans. B. Alan Wallace (Ithaca, NY: Snow Lion, 1998).

21. Karma Chagmé, *A Spacious Path to Freedom*, 82.

22. H.H. the Dalai Lama and Alexander Berzin, *The Gelug/Kagyü Tradition of Mahamudra* (Ithaca, NY: Snow Lion, 1997), 37–142; Karma Chagmé, *A Spacious Path to Freedom*, 80.

23. This citation is from the "Sems gnas pa'i thabs" section of his *Dge ldan bka' brgyud rin po che'i bka' srol phyag rgya chen po'i rtsa ba rgyas par bshad pa yang gsal sgron me* (photocopy in author's possession).

24. *Ratnameghasūtra*, cited in Śāntideva, *Śikṣāsamuccaya*, 68.

25. For a discussion of such techniques for realizing the primordial nature of awareness, see Karma Chagmé, *A Spacious Path to Freedom*, chs. 4–6, and Padmasambhava, *Natural Liberation*, 114–40.

26. For a fascinating account of this problem and its radical solution, see E. T. Whittaker, *A History of the Theories of Aether and Electricity, Modern Theories 1900–1926* (New York: Philosophical Library, 1954), ch. 3.

8. BEYOND IDOLATRY: THE RENAISSANCE OF A SPIRIT OF EMPIRICISM

1. Francis Bacon, *Novum Organum*, trans. and ed. P. Urbach and J. Gibson (Peru, IL: Open Court, 1994).

2. David Ritz Finkelstein, "Emptiness and Relativity," in *Buddhism and Science: Breaking New Ground*, ed. B. Alan Wallace (New York: Columbia University Press, 2003), 365–84.

3. Jeffrey Hopkins, *Meditation on Emptiness* (London: Wisdom, 1983), 296–304.

4. René Descartes, *Discourse on the Method; and Meditations on First Philosophy*, ed. David Weissman (New Haven: Yale University Press, 1996), *Meditations* 1, 2, 6.

5. S. B. Klein, "The Cognitive Neuroscience of Knowing One's Self," in *The Cognitive Neurosciences III*, ed. M. S. Gazzaniga (Cambridge, MA: MIT Press, 2004), 1077–1090; Owen Flanagan, *The Problem of the Soul: Two Visions of Mind and How to Reconcile Them* (New York: Basic Books, 2002); Charles Taylor, *Sources of the Self: The Making of the Modern Identity* (Cambridge, MA: Harvard University Press, 1989).

6. Steven Collins, *Selfless Persons: Imagery and Thought in Theravāda Buddhism* (London: Cambridge University Press, 1982).

7. Aristotle, *The Metaphysics*, trans. John H. McMahon (Buffalo, NY: Prometheus, 1991), 12.7; 1072b14.

8. Ibid., 12.7; 1073a4.

9. Albert Einstein, "Science and Religion," in *Out of My Later Years* (New York: Philosophical Library, 1950), 27.

10. Albert Einstein, "On Scientific Truth," In *Ideas and Opinions* (New York: Crown, 1954), 262.

11. John R. Searle, *The Rediscovery of the Mind* (Cambridge, MA: MIT Press, 1994), 90–91.

12. Daniel M. Wegner, *The Illusion of Conscious Will* (Cambridge, MA: MIT Press, 2003), 341–42.

13. B. Libet, C. A. Gleason, E. W. Wright, and D. K. Pearl, "Time of Conscious Intention to Act in Relation to Onset of Cerebral Activity (Readiness-Potential). The Unconscious Initiation of a Freely Voluntary Act." *Brain* 106 (3) (1983): 623–42.

14. Jack, Anthony I. and Philip Robbins, "Review of Wegner's *Illusion of Conscious Will*," *Behavioral and Brain Sciences* 27 (2004): 649–92.

15. Searle, *The Rediscovery of the Mind*, 76–77.

16. John R. Searle, *Consciousness and Language* (Cambridge: Cambridge University Press, 2002), 50.

17. Searle, *The Rediscovery of the Mind*, 3.

18. Paul C. W. Davies, "An Overview of the Contributions of John Archibald Wheeler," in *Science and Ultimate Reality: Quantum Theory, Cosmology and Complexity, Honoring John Wheeler's 90th Birthday*, ed. John D. Barrow, Paul C. W. Davies, and Charles L. Harper Jr. (Cambridge: Cambridge University Press, 2004), 5–6.

19. Ibid., 7.

20. *Prevention & Treatment*, Volume 1, Article 0002a, posted June 26, 1998. The full article may be viewed at: http://www.journals.apa.org/prevention/volume1/pre0010002a.html. A more recent and more comprehensive version of the argument, published in 2002, called "The Emperor's New Drugs: An Analysis of Antidepressant Medication Data Submitted to the U.S. Food and Drug Administration," can be accessed at: www.journals.apa.org/prevention/volume5/toc-jul15–02.html. For a broad, cultural perspective on the placebo effect in general, see Daniel E. Moerman, *Meaning, Medicine, and the "Placebo Effect"* (New York: Cambridge University Press, 2002).

21. Andrew F. Leuchter et al., "Changes in Brain Function of Depressed Subjects During Treatment with Placebo," *American Journal of Psychiatry* 159 (2002): 122–29.

22. Searle, *Consciousness and Language*, 34.

23. Antoine Lutz et al., "Long-Term Meditators Self-Induce High-Amplitude Gamma Synchrony During Mental Practice," *Proceedings of the National Academy of Sciences* 101, no. 46 (Nov. 16, 2004): 16369–16373. The full article can be found at: http://www.pnas.org/cgi/content/full/101/46/16369.

24. Edward J. Larson and Larry Witham, "Leading Scientists Still Reject God," *Nature* 394 (1998): 313.

25. René Descartes, *Principles of Philosophy*, Pt. 4, § 187, in *Oeuvres Philosophiques de Descartes*, trans. and ed. F. Alquié (Paris: Garnier Frères, 1973), 3:502n.

26. Werner Heisenberg, *Physics and Philosophy* (London: Penguin, 1989), 59; see also E. Schrödinger, *The Interpretation of Quantum Mechanics* (Woodbridge, CT: Ox Bow Press, 1995); H. D. Zeh, "There Are No Quantum Jumps, Nor Are There Particles," *Physics Letters* A172 (1993): 189–92; P. C. W. Davies, "Particles Do Not Exist," in *Quantum Theory of Gravity*, ed. S. M. Christiansen (New York: Adam Hilger, 1984); Michel Bitbol, *Schrödinger's Philosophy of Quantum Mechanics* (New York: Kluwer, 1995).

27. P. M. Haman, *Energy, Force and Matter: The Conceptual Development of Nineteenth Century Physics* (Cambridge: Cambridge University Press, 1982), 43.

28. Richard P. Feynman, R. B. Leighton, and M. Sands, *The Feynman Lectures on Physics* (Cambridge, MA: MIT Press, 1965), sec. 4–2.

29. Tim Folger, "Does the Universe Exist if We're Not Looking?" *Discover* 23, no. 6 (June 2002). For the full article, see: http://www.discover.com/issues/jun-02/features/featuniverse/; Anton Zeilinger, "Why the Quantum? 'It' from 'Bit'? A Participatory Universe? Three Far-Reaching Challenges from John Archibald Wheeler and Their Relation to Experiment," in *Science and Ultimate Reality: Quantum Theory, Cosmology and Complexity, Honoring John Wheeler's 90th Birthday*, ed. John D. Barrow, Paul C. W. Davies, and Charles L. Harper Jr. (Cambridge: Cambridge University Press, 2004) 201–20; Jacob D. Bekenstein, "Information in the Holographic Universe—Theoretical Results About Black Holes Suggest That the Universe Could Be Like a Gigantic Hologram," *Scientific American* (August 2003); David Bohm, *Thought as a System* (London: Routledge, 1994); David Bohm, *Wholeness and the Implicate Order* (London: Routledge, 1995).

30. John Archibald Wheeler, "Beyond the Black Hole," in *Some Strangeness in the Proportion: A Centennial Symposium to Celebrate the Achievements of Albert Einstein*, ed. Harry Woolf (Reading, MA: Addison-Wesley, 1980), 356; John Archibald Wheeler, "The 'Past' and the 'Delayed-Choice' Double-Slit Experiment," in *Mathematical Foundations of Quantum Theory*, ed. A. R. Marlow (New York: Academic Press, 1978).

31. Finkelstein, "Emptiness and Relativity," 366.

32. Michel Bitbol, "Materialism, Stances, and Open-Mindedness," in *Images of Empiricism: Essays on Science and Stances, with a Reply from Bas van Fraassen*, ed. Bradley Monton (Oxford: Oxford University Press, in press).

33. Michael Lockwood, *Mind, Brain and the Quantum* (Oxford: Basil Blackwell, 1989), 20.

34. Hilary Putnam, *The Many Faces of Realism* (La Salle: Open Court, 1987); *Realism with a Human Face*, ed. James Conant (Cambridge, MA: Harvard University Press, 1990); "Replies and Comments," *Erkenntnis* 34, no. 3 (1991).

35. E. R. Harrison, *Cosmology: The Science of the Universe*, 2nd ed. (Cambridge: Cambridge University Press, 2000); George F. R. Ellis, "True Complexity and Its Associated Ontology," in *Science and Ultimate Reality: Quantum Theory, Cosmology and Complexity, Honoring John Wheeler's 90th Birthday*, ed. John D. Barrow, Paul

C. W. Davies, and Charles L. Harper Jr. (Cambridge: Cambridge University Press, 2004), 607–36.

36. Robert B. Laughlin, *A Different Universe: Reinventing Physics from the Bottom Down* (Basic Books, 2005), 31, 55.

37. Ibid., 14.

38. George F. R. Ellis, "Physics, Complexity and Causality," *Nature* 435 (2005): 743; "Physics and the Real World," *Physics Today* 58 (2005): 49–55.

39. Finkelstein, "Emptiness and Relativity," 367–68.

40. Andre Linde, "Inflation, Quantum Cosmology and the Anthropic Principle," in *Science and Ultimate Reality: Quantum Theory, Cosmology and Complexity, Honoring John Wheeler's 90th Birthday*, ed. John D. Barrow, Paul C. W. Davies, and Charles L. Harper Jr. (Cambridge: Cambridge University Press, 2004), 426–58.

41. Finkelstein, "Emptiness and Relativity," 380.

42. For this discussion, I am indebted to the wonderful insights expressed in Michel Bitbol's essay "Materialism, Stances, and Open-Mindedness," and to our correspondence concerning these issues.

43. Laughlin, *A Different Universe*, 55.

44. H. H. the Dalai Lama, *The Universe in a Single Atom: The Convergence of Science and Spirituality* (New York: Morgan Road, 2005).

45. Thomas S. Kuhn, *The Structure of Scientific Revolutions*, 2nd ed. (Chicago: University of Chicago Press, 1970).

46. Laughlin, *A Different Universe*, 13.

47. Francisco Varela and Jeremy Hayward, eds., *Gentle Bridges: Conversations with the Dalai Lama on the Sciences of Mind*, 2nd ed. (Boston: Shambhala, 1992), 37.

48. M. Kline, *Mathematics: The Loss of Certainty* (New York: Oxford University Press, 1980), 59.

49. K. C. Cole, *The Hole in the Universe: How Scientists Peered Over the Edge of Emptiness and Found Everything* (New York: Harcourt, 2001), 244.

50. Basil Hiley, "Vacuum or Holomovement," in *The Philosophy of Vacuum*, ed. Simon Saunders and Harvey R. Brown (New York: Oxford University Press, 1991); H. Atmanspacher, "Mind and Matter as Asymptotically Disjoint, Inequivalent Representations with Broken Time-Reversal Symmetry," *BioSystems* 68 (2003): 19–30; Henry P. Stapp, *Mind, Matter, and Quantum Mechanics* (New York: Springer, 2004); M. B. Menski, "Concept of Consciousness in the Context of Quantum Mechanics," *Physics—Uspekhi* 48 (4) (2005): 389–409; Mark Stuckey, Michael Silberstein, and Michael Cifone, "Reversing the Arrow of Explanation in the Relational Blockworld: Why Temporal Becoming, the Dynamical Brain and the External World Are All in 'in the Mind,'" in *Endophysics, Time, Quantum and the Subjective*, ed. R. Buccheri et al. (London: World Scientific Publishing, 2005), 207–30.

51. Cole, *The Hole in the Universe*, 177–78.

52. Düdjom Lingpa, *The Vajra Essence: From the Matrix of Pure Appearances and Primordial Consciousness, a Tantra on the Self-Originating Nature of Existence*, trans. B. Alan Wallace (Alameda, CA: Mirror of Wisdom, 2004), 255.

53. Ibid., 251.

54. Ibid., 210–12.

55. Padmasambhava, *Natural Liberation: Padmasambhava's Teachings on the Six Bardos*, commentary by Gyaltrul Rinpoche; trans. B. Alan Wallace (Boston: Wisdom, 1998), 62.

56. I. P. Sheldon-Williams, trans. and comm., *Periphyseon (De divisione naturae)*, Book 2 (Dublin: Dublin Institute for Advanced Studies, 1968–72), 143–45 (589B–C).

57. H. Lawrence Bond, trans., *Nicholas of Cusa: Selected Spiritual Writings* (New York: Paulist Press, 1997), *On Seeking God (De quaerendo Deum* 1445), 230.

58. Ibid., 251.

59. Robert K. C. Forman, ed., *The Problem of Pure Consciousness: Mysticism and Philosophy* (New York: Oxford University Press, 1990).

60. William James, *Pragmatism* (Cambridge: Harvard University Press, 1975).

61. Henry P. Stapp, *Mind, Matter, and Quantum Mechanics* (Berlin: Springer, 1993); Basil J. Hiley, "Quantum Mechanics and the Relation Between Mind and Matter," in *Brain, Mind and Physics*, ed. P. Pylkkänen et al. (Helsinki: IOS Press, 1997), 37–53; Laughlin, *A Different Universe*.

62. Laughlin, *A Different Universe*, 14.

63. Ibid.,116.

64. B. Van Fraassen, *The Empirical Stance* (New Haven: Yale University Press, 2002), 61.

65. Nick Herbert, *Quantum Reality: Beyond the New Physics* (Garden City, NY: Anchor Press/Doubleday, 1985), 248.

BIBLIOGRAPHY

Aristotle. *Nicomachean Ethics*. Trans. Terence Irwin. Indianapolis: Hackett, 1985.

Aronson, Harvey B. *Love and Sympathy in Theravāda Buddhism*. Delhi: Motilal Banarsidass, 1980.

Augustine. *The Confessions*. Trans. Maria Boulding. Hyde Park, NY: New City Press, 1997.

——. *The Free Choice of the Will*. Trans. Francis E. Tourscher. Philadelphia: Peter Reilly, 1937.

——. *Letters 100–155 (Epistolae)*. Trans. Roland Teske. Hyde Park, NY: New City Press, 2003.

Banerjee, Nikunja Vihari, ed. *The Dhammapada*. New Delhi: Munshiram Manoharlal, 1989.

Bareau, A. *Les Sectes Bouddhiques du Petit Véhicule*. Paris: EFEO, 1955.

Batchelor, Stephen. *Buddhism Without Beliefs: A Contemporary Guide to Awakening*. New York: Riverhead, 1997.

Bond, H. L., trans. *Nicholas of Cusa: Selected Spiritual Writings*. New York: Paulist Press, 1997.

Boorstin, Daniel J. *The Discoverers: A History of Man's Search to Know His World and Himself*. New York: Vintage, 1985.

Bronkhorst, J. *Why Is There Philosophy in India*. Amsterdam: Royal Netherlands Academy of Arts and Sciences, 1999.

Buber, Martin. *I and Thou*. Trans. Walter Kaufmann. 1937; reprint, New York: Touchstone, 1996.

Burnaby, John. *Amor Dei: A Study of the Religion of St. Augustine*. 1938; reprint, Norwich: Canterbury Press, 1991.

Buswell Jr., Robert E. and Robert M. Gimello, eds. *Paths to Liberation: The Mārga and Its Transformations in Buddhist Thought*. Honolulu: University of Hawaii Press, 1992.

Butler, Dom Cuthbert. *Western Mysticism: The Teaching of Augustine, Gregory, and Bernard on Contemplation and the Contemplative Life.* 3rd ed. London: Constable, 1967.

Cabezón, José Ignacio. *Buddhism and Language: A Study of Indo-Tibetan Scholasticism.* Albany: State University of New York Press, 1994.

Chadwick, Owen, trans. and ed. *The Conferences of Cassian in Western Asceticism.* Philadelphia: Westminster Press, 1958.

Chalmers, David J. *Conscious Mind: In Search of a Fundamental Theory.* New York: Oxford University Press, 1996.

Chang, G. C. C., trans. and ed. *The Hundred Thousand Songs of Milarepa.* Boulder, CO: Shambhala, 1962.

Chene, R. "Is Every Mediation Multicultural?" In conference handbook, Northern California Mediation Association, March 18, 2000.

Cole, K. C. *The Hole in the Universe: How Scientists Peered Over the Edge of Emptiness and Found Everything.* New York: Harcourt, 2001.

Crick, F. and C. Koch. "Towards a Neurobiological Theory of Consciousness" In *The Nature of Consciousness: Philosophical Debates*, ed. N. Block, O. Flanagan, and G. Güzeldere, 277–92. Cambridge, MA: MIT Press, 1997.

H. H. the Dalai Lama. *Dzogchen: The Heart Essence of the Great Perfection.* Trans. Geshe Thupten Jinpa and Richard Barron. Ithaca, NY: Snow Lion, 2000.

——. *Ethics for the New Millennium.* New York: Riverhead, 1999.

——. *Transcendent Wisdom: A Teaching on the Wisdom Section of Shantideva's Guide to the Bodhisattva Way of Life.* Trans., ed., and annot. B. Alan Wallace. Ithaca, NY: Snow Lion, 1994.

H. H. the Dalai Lama and Alexander Berzin. *The Gelug/Kagyü Tradition of Mahamudra.* Ithaca, NY: Snow Lion, 1997.

H. H. the Dalai Lama and Howard C. Cutler, M.D. *The Art of Happiness: A Handbook for Living.* New York: Riverhead, 1998.

Damasio, Antonio R. *The Feeling of What Happens: Body and Emotion in the Making of Consciousness.* New York: Harcourt, 1999.

Danziger, K. "The History of Introspection Reconsidered." *Journal of the History of the Behavioral Sciences* 16 (1980): 241–62.

Davies, Paul C. W. "An Overview of the Contributions of John Archibald Wheeler." In *Science and Ultimate Reality: Quantum Theory, Cosmology and Complexity, Honoring John Wheeler's 90th Birthday*, ed. John D. Barrow, Paul C. W. Davies, and Charles L. Harper Jr. Cambridge: Cambridge University Press, 2004, 3–26.

Dennett, Daniel C. *Consciousness Explained.* Boston: Little, Brown, 1991.

Dreyfus, B. G. *Recognizing Reality: Dharmakīrti's Philosophy and Its Tibetan Interpretations.* Delhi: Sri Satguru, 1997.

Duclow, Donald F. "Divine Nothingness and Self-Creation in John Scotus Eriugena." *The Journal of Religion* 57, no. 2 (April 1977).

Düdjom Lingpa. *The Vajra Essence: From the Matrix of Pure Appearances and Primordial Consciousness, a Tantra on the Self-Originating Nature of Existence.* Trans. B. Alan Wallace. Alameda, CA: Mirror of Wisdom, 2004.

Ekman, Paul, Richard J. Davidson, Matthieu Ricard, and B. Alan Wallace. "Buddhist and Psychological Perspectives on Emotions and Well-Being." *Current Directions in Psychology* 14, no. 2 (2005): 59–63.

Eriugena, John Scotus. *Periphyseon (De divisione naturae)*. Ed. H. J. Floss. Migne *Patrologia latina* 122, 680D–81A. Trans. Donald F. Duclow. Ridgewood, NJ: Gregg Press, 1965.

Evans-Wentz, W. Y., ed. *The Tibetan Book of the Great Liberation*. London: Oxford University Press, 1968.

Feynman, Richard. *The Character of Physical Law*. Cambridge, MA: MIT Press, 1983.

Forman, Robert K. C., ed. *The Problem of Pure Consciousness: Mysticism and Philosophy*. New York: Oxford University Press, 1990.

Freud, S. *Civilization and Its Discontents*. Trans. and ed. James Strachey. New York: Norton, 1961.

Garfield, Jay L., trans. *The Fundamental Wisdom of the Middle Way: Nāgārjuna's Mūlamadhyamakakārikā*. New York: Oxford University Press, 1995.

Gendün-drup (dge 'dun grub). *Ornament of Reasoning, a Great Treatise on Valid Cognition (tshad ma'i bstan bcos chen po rigs pa'i rgyan)*. Mundgod, India: Loling Press, 1985.

Genz, Henning. *Nothingness: The Science of Empty Space*. Trans. by Karin Heusch. Cambridge, MA: Perseus, 1999.

Gethin, R. M. L. *The Buddhist Path to Awakening*. Oxford: Oneworld, 2001.

Gnoli, R., ed. *The Pramāṇavārttikam of Dharmakīrti*. Rome: Serie Orientale Roma 23, 1960.

Goleman, Daniel, ed. *Healing Emotions: Conversations with the Dalai Lama on Mindfulness, Emotions, and Health*. Boston: Shambhala, 1997.

Gómez, L. "Measuring the Immeasurable: Reflections on Unreasonable Reasoning." In *Buddhist Theology: Critical Reflections by Contemporary Buddhist Scholars*, ed. Roger R. Jackson and John Makransky. Surrey, England: Curzon, 1999, 367–85.

Guenther, Herbert V. and Leslie S. Kawamura. *Mind in Buddhist Psychology*. Emeryville, CA: Dharma, 1975.

Hanh, Thich Nhat. *Living Buddha, Living Christ*. New York: Riverhead, 1997.

Harvey, Peter. *The Selfless Mind: Personality, Consciousness, and Nirvana in Early Buddhism*. Surrey, England: Curzon, 1995.

Heisenberg, Werner. *Physics and Beyond: Encounters and Conversations*. New York: Harper and Row, 1971.

——. *Physics and Philosophy: The Revolution in Modern Science*. New York: Harper and Row, 1962.

Holmes, K. H. and K. Holmes. *The Changeless Continuity*. 2nd ed. Eskdalemuir, Scotland: Karma Drubgyud Darjay Ling, 1985.

Hopkins, Jeffrey. *Meditation on Emptiness*. London: Wisdom, 1983.

Huxley, Aldous. *The Perennial Philosophy*. London: Chatto & Windus, 1946.

Jack, A. and A. Roepstorff, eds. *Trusting the Subject? Journal of Consciousness Studies* (special issue). Exeter: Imprint Academic, 2003.

Jackson, R. R. "In Search of a Postmodern Middle." In *Buddhist Theology: Critical Reflections by Contemporary Buddhist Scholars*, ed. Roger R. Jackson and John Makransky. Surrey, England: Curzon, 1999, 215–46.

———. *Is Enlightenment Possible?: Dharmakīrti and rGyal tshab rje on Knowledge, Rebirth, No-Self, and Liberation*. Ithaca, NY: Snow Lion, 1993.

James, William. *Essays in Radical Empiricism*. 1912; reprint, Cambridge, MA: Harvard University Press, 1976.

———. *Essays in Religion and Morality*. Cambridge, MA: Harvard University Press, 1989.

———. "The Notion of Consciousness." In *The Writings of William James*, ed. J. J. McDermott. 1905; reprint, Chicago: University of Chicago Press, 1977.

———. *The Principles of Psychology*. 1890; reprint, New York: Dover, 1950.

———. *Some Problems of Philosophy: A Beginning of an Introduction to Philosophy*. London: Longmans, Green, 1911.

———. *The Varieties of Religious Experience: A Study in Human Nature*. New York: Longmans, Green, 1902.

———. "A World of Pure Experience." In *The Writings of William James*, ed. John J. McDermott. 1912; reprint, Chicago: University of Chicago Press, 1977, 194–214.

Jamgön Kongtrul Lodrö Tayé. *Myriad Worlds: Buddhist Cosmology in Abhidharma, Kālacakra, and Dzog-chen*. Trans. and ed. the International Translation Committee. Ithaca, NY: Snow Lion, 1995.

Kalupahana, David J. *The Principles of Buddhist Psychology*. Albany: State University of New York Press, 1987.

Kamalaśīla. *First Bhāvanākrama*. Ed. G. Tucci. In *Minor Buddhist Texts, Part II*. Rome: Istituto italiano per il Medio ed Estremo Oriente, 1958.

Kant, Immanuel. *Metaphysical Foundations of Natural Science*. Trans. James Ellington. 1786; reprint, Indianapolis: Bobbs-Merrill, 1970.

Karma Chagmé. *A Spacious Path to Freedom: Practical Instructions on the Union of Mahāmudrā and Atiyoga*. Commentary by Gyatrul Rinpoche. Trans. B. Alan Wallace. Ithaca, NY: Snow Lion, 1998.

Kasser, Tim. *The High Price of Materialism*. Boston: MIT Press, 2002.

Klein, Anne C. "Mental Concentration and the Unconditioned: A Buddhist Case for Unmediated Experience." In *Paths to Liberation: The Mārga and Its Transformations in Buddhist Thought*, ed. Robert E. Buswell Jr. and Robert M. Gimello. Delhi: Motilal Banarsidass, 1992, 269–308.

Klein, Anne C. *Path to the Middle: Oral Mādhyamika Philosophy in Tibet*. Albany: State University of New York Press, 1994.

Kline, M. *Mathematics: The Loss of Certainty*. New York: Oxford University Press, 1980.

Kuhn, Thomas S. *The Structure of Scientific Revolutions*. 2nd ed. Chicago: University of Chicago Press, 1970.

LaBerge, Stephen. "Lucid Dreaming and the Yoga of the Dream State: A Psycho-physiological Perspective." In *Buddhism and Science: Breaking New Ground*, ed. B. Alan Wallace. New York: Columbia University Press, 2003, 233–58.

LaBerge, Stephen and Howard Rheingold. *Exploring the World of Lucid Dreaming*. New York: Ballantine, 1990.

Lamrimpa, Gen. *Calming the Mind: Tibetan Buddhist Teachings on the Cultivation of Meditative Quiescence*. Trans. B. Alan Wallace. Ithaca, NY: Snow Lion, 1995.

——. *Realizing Emptiness: Madhyamaka Insight Meditation*. Trans. B. Alan Wallace. Ithaca, NY: Snow Lion, 2002.

Lati Rinbochay. *Mind in Tibetan Buddhism*. Trans. and ed. Elizabeth Napper. Valois, France: Gabriel/Snow Lion, 1981.

Loy, David. *Nonduality: A Study in Comparative Philosophy*. New Haven: Yale University Press, 1988.

Maréchal, Joseph, S.J. *Studies in the Psychology of the Mystics*. Trans. Algar Thorold. London: Burns, Oates, & Washbourne, 1927.

Matt, Daniel C. *"Ayin*: The Concept of Nothingness in Jewish Mysticism." In *The Problem of Pure Consciousness: Mysticism and Philosophy*, ed. Robert K.C. Forman. New York: Oxford University Press, 1990.

——. *The Essential Kabbalah: The Heart of Jewish Mysticism*. San Francisco: HarperSanFrancisco, 1995.

McDermott, John J., ed. *The Writings of William James: A Comprehensive Edition*. Chicago: University of Chicago Press, 1977.

McGinn, Bernard and John Meyendorff, eds. *Christian Spirituality: Origins to the Twelfth Century*. New York: Crossroad, 1985.

Mullin, Glenn H., trans. *Tsongkhapa's Six Yogas of Naropa*. Ithaca, NY: Snow Lion, 1996.

Nagel, T. *The View from Nowhere*. New York: Oxford University Press, 1986.

Ñāṇamoli, B. *The Life of the Buddha According to the Pali Canon*. Kandy, Sri Lanka: Buddhist Publication Society, 1992.

Oparin, Aleksandr. *The Origin of Life*. Trans. Sergius Morgulis. New York: Macmillan, 1938.

Padmasambhava. *Natural Liberation: Padmasambhava's Teachings on the Six Bardos*. Commentary by Gyatrul Rinpoche. Trans. B. Alan Wallace. Boston: Wisdom, 1998.

Patton, K.C. "Juggling Torches: Why We Still Need Comparative Religion." In *A Magic Still Dwells: Comparative Religion in the Postmodern Age,* ed. K.C. Patton and B. C. Rav. Berkeley: University of California Press, 2000, 153–71.

Patton, K.C. and B. C. Rav, eds. *A Magic Still Dwells: Comparative Religion in the Postmodern Age*. Berkeley: University of California Press, 2000.

Pieper, Josef. *Happiness and Contemplation*. Trans. Richard and Clara Winston. Chicago: Henry Regnery, 1966.

Plato. *Phaedo*. Trans. Robin Waterfield. New York: Oxford University Press, 2002.

Posner, M.I. *Chronometric Exploration of Mind*. Hillsdale, NJ: Lawrence Erlbaum Associates, 1978.

Putnam, Hilary. *Realism with a Human Face*. Ed. James Conant. Cambridge, MA: Harvard University Press, 1990.

——. "Replies and Comments." *Erkenntnis* 34, no. 3 (1991).

Rabten, Geshe. *The Mind and Its Functions*. Trans. Stephen Batchelor. Mt. Pèlerin, Switz.: Tharpa Choeling, 1979.

Rahula, Walpola. *What the Buddha Taught*. New York: Grove Weidenfeld, 1974.

Robinson, R.H. *The Buddhist Religion*. 1st ed. Belmont, CA: Dickenson, 1970.

Śāntideva. *A Guide to the Bodhisattva Way of Life.* Trans. Vesna A. Wallace and B. Alan Wallace. Ithaca, NY: Snow Lion, 1997.

——. *Śikṣāsamuccaya: A Compendium of Buddhist Doctrine.* Ed. P. D. Vaidya. Darbhanga, India: Mithila Institute, 1961.

Schrödinger, E. *Mind and Matter.* Cambridge: Cambridge University Press, 1958.

Searle, John R. *Consciousness and Language.* Cambridge: Cambridge University Press, 2002.

——. *The Rediscovery of the Mind.* Cambridge, MA: MIT Press, 1994.

Sharf, R. H. "Buddhist Modernism and the Rhetoric of Meditative Experiences." *Numen* 42 (1995): 228–83.

——. "Experience." In *Critical Terms for Religious Studies,* ed. Mark C. Taylor. Chicago: University of Chicago Press, 1998, 94–116.

Shastri D., ed. *Tattvasaṃgraha.* Varanasi: Bauddhabharati, 1968.

Siegfried, T. *The Bit and the Pendulum: From Quantum Computing to M Theory—The New Physics of Information.* New York: Wiley, 2000.

Snyder, C. R. and Shane J. Lopez, eds. *Handbook of Positive Psychology.* New York: Oxford University Press, 2002.

Sonam, Ruth. *Atisha's Lamp for the Path.* Commentary by Geshe Sonam Rinchen. Ithaca, NY: Snow Lion, 1997.

——, trans. *Yogic Deeds of Bodhisattvas: Gyel-tsap on Āryadeva's Four Hundred.* Commentary by Geshe Sonam Rinchen. Ithaca, NY: Snow Lion, 1994.

Stuckey, Mark, Michael Silberstein, and Michael Cifone. "Reversing the Arrow of Explanation in the Relational Blockworld: Why Temporal Becoming, the Dynamical Brain, and the External World Are All 'in the Mind.'" In *Endophysics, Time, Quantum, and the Subjective,* ed. R. Buccheri et al. London: World Scientific Publishing, 2005, 207–30.

Thera, Nyanaponika. *The Heart of Buddhist Meditation.* New York: Samuel Weiser, 1973.

Thera, Soma. *The Way of Mindfulness: The Satipaṭṭhāna Sutta and Commentary.* Kandy, Sri Lanka: Buddhist Publication Society, 1975.

Tillemans, T. "Indian and Tibetan Mādhyamikas on *Mānasapratyakśa.*" *Tibet Journal* 14, no. 1 (1989): 70–85.

——. *Scripture, Logic, Language: Essays on Dharmakīrti and His Tibetan Successors.* Boston: Wisdom, 1999.

Tsongkhapa. *Byang chub lam rim chen mo.* Dharamsala, India: Tibetan Cultural Printing Press, n.d.

——. *The Great Treatise on the Stages of the Path to Enlightenment.* Vol. 3. Ithaca, NY: Snow Lion, 2002.

Vajirañāṇa, Paravahera. *Buddhist Meditation in Theory and Practice.* Kuala Lumpur, Malaysia: Buddhist Missionary Society, 1975.

Van Fraassen, B. *The Empirical Stance.* New Haven: Yale University Press, 2002.

Van Lommel, Pim, Ruud van Wees, Vincent Meyers, and Ingrid Elfferich. "Near-Death Experience in Survivors of Cardiac Arrest: A Prospective Study in the Netherlands." *The Lancet* 358 (2001): 2039–45.

Varela, F. J. "Neurophenomenology: A Methodological Remedy for the Hard Problem." *Journal of Consciousness Studies* 3, no. 4 (1996): 330–49.

Vasubandhu. *Abhidharmakośabhāṣyam*. French trans. Louis de La Vallée Poussin. English trans. Leo M. Pruden. Berkeley: Asian Humanities Press, 1991.

Waldron, William S. "Common Ground, Common Cause: Buddhism and Science on the Afflictions of Identity." In *Buddhism and Science: Breaking New Ground*, ed. B. Alan Wallace. New York: Columbia University Press, 2003, 145–91.

Wallace, B. Alan. *The Attention Revolution: Unlocking the Power of the Focused Mind*. Boston: Wisdom, 2006.

——. *Balancing the Mind: A Tibetan Buddhist Approach to Refining Attention*. Ithaca, NY: Snow Lion, 2005.

——. "Buddhism and Science." In *The Oxford Handbook of Religion and Science*, ed. Philip Clayton. New York: Oxford University Press, 2006.

——, ed. *Buddhism and Science: Breaking New Ground*. New York: Columbia University Press, 2003.

——. *Buddhism with an Attitude: The Tibetan Seven-Point Mind-Training*. Ithaca, NY: Snow Lion, 2001.

——. "The Buddhist Tradition of *Śamatha*: Methods for Refining and Examining Consciousness." *Journal of Consciousness Studies* 6, no. 2–3 (1999): 175–87.

——. *Choosing Reality: A Buddhist View of Physics and the Mind*. Ithaca, NY: Snow Lion, 1996.

——. "Energy Dynamics." *Life Positive* (Jan. 2006).

——. *The Four Immeasurables: Cultivating a Boundless Heart*. Rev. ed. Ithaca, NY: Snow Lion, 2004.

——. *Genuine Happiness: Meditation as the Path to Fulfillment*. Hoboken, NJ: Wiley, 2005.

——. "The Intersubjective Worlds of Science and Religion." In *Science, Religion, and the Human Experience*, ed. James Proctor. New York: Oxford University Press, 2005.

——. *The Taboo of Subjectivity: Toward a New Science of Consciousness*. New York: Oxford University Press, 2000.

——. *Tibetan Buddhism from the Ground Up*. With Steven Wilhelm. Boston: Wisdom, 1993.

——. "Vacuum States of Consciousness: A Tibetan Buddhist View." In *Buddhist Thought and Applied Psychology: Transcending the Boundaries*, ed. D. K. Nauriyal. London: Routledge-Curzon, 2006.

Walshe, M. O. C., trans. *Meister Eckhart: Sermons and Treatises*. Vols. I–III. Longmead: Element Books, 1979, 1987.

Watson, John. *Behaviorism*. 1913; reprint, New York: Norton, 1970.

Wayman, Alex and Hideko, trans. *The Lion's Road of Queen Śrīmālā*. Delhi: Motilal Banarsidass, 1990.

Weinberg, S. *The First Three Minutes: A Modern View of the Origin of the Universe*. New York: Basic Books, 1988.

Whittaker, E. T. *A History of the Theories of Aether and Electricity, Modern Theories 1900–1926*. New York: Philosophical Library, 1954.

Williams, Paul. *Mahāyāna Buddhism: The Doctrinal Foundations*. London: Routledge, 1989.

——. "Out of My Head." *The Tablet* 5 (Aug. 2000).

Wilson, Edward O. *Consilience: The Unity of Knowledge*. New York: Knopf, 1998.

Woods, James Haughton. *The Yoga System of Patañjali*. Reprint, Delhi: Motilal Banarsidass, 1983.

Zeilinger, Anton. "Why the Quantum? 'It' from 'Bit'? A Participatory Universe? Three Far-Reaching Challenges from John Archibald Wheeler and Their Relation to Experiment." In *Science and Ultimate Reality: Quantum Theory, Cosmology and Complexity, Honoring John Wheeler's 90th Birthday*, ed. John D. Barrow, Paul C. W. Davies, and Charles L. Harper Jr. Cambridge: Cambridge University Press, 2004, 201–20.

INDEX